10TH ANNIVERSARY

The

MIRACLE
KIDNEY
CLEANSE

10TH ANNIVERSARY EDITION

The MIRACLE KIDNEY CLEANSE

The All-Natural, At-Home Flush to Purify Your Body

LAUREN FELTS

Published by:
Ulysses Press
PO Box 3440
Berkeley, CA 94703
www.ulyssespress.com

ISBN: 978-1-64604-704-8
Library of Congress Control Number: 2024934569

Printed in the United States

10 9 8 7 6 5 4 3 2 1

Managing editor: Claire Chun
Proofreader: Laurie Dunne
Index: S4Carlisle Publishing Services
Front cover design: Winnie Liu
Artwork from shutterstock.com: cover © mama_mia_CMYK; page 97
butterfly pose © Roman Zherdytskyi, downward dog pose © Roi Brooks,
upward dog pose © Guryanov Andrey, saddle pose © nanka, sphinx pose ©
Christopher Edwin Nuzzaco, child's pose © Guryanov Andrey, straddle pose
© Denisa V, knee-to-head forward fold pose © Guryanov Andrey; page 98
full forward pose © Guryanov Andrey, runner's stretch © Artur Bogacki;
page 99 kidney illustration © snapgalleria

CONTENTS

FOREWORD

If you have picked up this book and are reading these words, I bet you are wondering how you will manage to read an entire book about the kidneys.

While I will admit that the topic of the kidneys, on the surface, may seem about as interesting as watching a dental exam, I will prove to you otherwise if you have the guts to read a little bit farther. My goal is to give you lots of juicy information about how to take care of your kidneys and how important they are to your health, but it will not do you or me any good if I cannot get you to actually read this book. Therefore, I pledge to do my darndest to make this book as fun and lighthearted as it is informative and effective. Scout's honor.

The kidneys. How in the world did I get so interested in the kidneys that I wrote a book about cleansing them? To tell you the truth, I have done a lot of cleansing. I've cleansed my liver and my intestines, I've cleansed heavy metals, candida, and toxins in general, and the kidneys were my last stop on the line. And why, you may ask? Unlike other cleansing protocols, a standard kidney cleanse had not been developed, and the kidneys' role in the body remains underappreciated for its ability to rapidly transform health.

Guess what happened when I started cleansing my kidneys? Those nagging symptoms that had not cleared with other forms of cleansing or with diet changes alone finally dissipated. I am not saying that cleansing your kidneys will make you completely symptom- and disease-free, but I am saying that it is essential to regaining good health. Yes, you definitely should incorporate other cleanses, but the bottom line is that you have to cleanse your kidneys as well.

The great part about committing to this program is that it will target the root of your health issues and symptoms, and also help you make drastic changes in the way you feel and live. I developed this cleanse not just to get rid of symptoms temporarily, but to foster real change at the core. This cleanse will provide you with all the tools you need to get out of the vicious cycle of quick fixes and chronic ailments and into a space where you are building a platform for radiant health. We all need a good kick in the butt to get us motivated and out of our comfort zone. And here I am, your big kick in the butt.

Now, let's get cleansing!

INTRODUCTION

The kidneys, which sit right above the pelvic bone, are positioned on either side of the spinal column. Bean-shaped and each about the size of a computer mouse, the kidneys are involved in a multitude of functions that go far beyond urine generation. What I learned about the power of the kidneys and their influence over the body completely changed my outlook on health. As soon as I started addressing the kidneys holistically, the rest of my body system began to fall into place. Chronic symptoms such as low back pain, hair loss, fatigue, bone loss, and reproductive challenges started to reverse themselves, and so many of those nasty ailments that seem to plague so many of us dissipated. It was as if I had discovered the hidden key, the missing link that could offer new solutions for tapping into radiant health.

The kidneys' connection and proximity to the bladder and adrenal glands are key to their holistic role in the body. It is due partly to this physical location that they are seen as the ministers of power in Chinese medicine, providing both the nourishing and stabilizing qualities that are needed for life as well as greatly influencing body functions as a whole.

In the Western world, the kidneys are recognized for their ability to concentrate urine and maintain homeostasis, or equilibrium, while also playing a less prominent role in vitamin D synthesis and red blood cell generation. In contrast, in the Eastern world, energetic health begins and ends with the kidney force, giving rise to the kidneys' reputation as the root of vital destiny. The real intrigue about this very delicate yet powerful organ is its ability not only to control the fine balance of our system, but also to influence our innate essence of youthfulness, vigor, and "life fire." Therefore, this book does more than just look at the mechanics of the kidneys, what they do, and how to get them functioning optimally—it also delves into the "X factor," which holds the real secrets to amazing health. It will help you work toward cleaning your proverbial house and creating an indestructible foundation, which will allow you to tap into the power needed to reignite your life fire and take back the health and energy of your early years.

The concept of cleansing is just starting to emerge in our daily vernacular, as the prevalence of symptoms and diagnoses is no longer regarded as aberrant, but rather as expected. Although cleansing may be completely new to you, it will shortly become a part of your health routine, matching the comfort level you might have with teeth cleaning, haircuts, and eye checkups. The world is changing, becoming more toxic, and the human body, as miraculous and fined-tuned as it is, was just not built for this type of environment. As an inherent desire to care for and protect the body kicks in, we ultimately look to our intuitive knowledge of health care: reduce toxic exposure, eat clean food, exercise, reduce stress, and cleanse.

This book is the first step in taking back your health, regardless of whether you are dealing with chronic disease or kidney dysfunction or are in perfect health. It is intended to educate, inspire, and direct you toward making key changes in your health, specifically in the health of your kidneys; it is not meant as a cure. Through the kidney cleanse protocol, along with dietary changes and steps to living a toxin-free life, you will have all the tools necessary to jump-start and ignite your path to a disease-free life full of vitality.

WHY IS IT SO IMPORTANT TO CLEANSE THE KIDNEYS?

Most people do not address kidney health or even think about the kidneys until there is something seriously wrong with them, but this very important organ pair deserves lots of love and attention. I contend that the kidneys are of prime importance, often acting as the missing link in the body-health connection. The problem is that they are often thought as the last stop in the body, merely a filter for concentrating urine, and are taken care of only in acute or chronic conditions, not when they are beginning to undergo stress.

This book is not simply a guide for dealing with acute kidney disorders, but a first stop in your journey toward superior health and vitality. In a world where chronic disease, nagging symptoms, and less-than-optimal body functioning are pervasive, I believe that the lack of attention given to the kidneys is partly to blame. This book can establish that link and create a foundation on which to build a blueprint for long-lasting health. The body was engineered not just to get by, but to excel and perform at levels far beyond what it is likely functioning at today. Ready to see how well you can perform?

HOW IS THIS APPROACH DIFFERENT?

On delving into the realm of health and wellness, I found that the integration of Western and Eastern practices is essential in uncovering the mysteries of our bodies. While the Western model excels at a biochemical level, the Eastern model is unparalleled at an energetic and integrated level. Fortunately, in this day and age we have been able to blend the two, reaching new levels of health and preventive care. I believe the two models are not meant to stand alone, but to act in unison, playing off each other like instruments in an orchestra. Together, they can address the human form as a whole rather than analyze it piecemeal and risk missing key aspects.

The best way that I can communicate the differences between these two methods of medical practice is that the Western model is like algebra, ideal for left-brain thinkers because it focuses on concrete facts, and the Eastern model is like geometry, ideal for right-brain thinkers because it requires abstract thought and visualization. Western medicine concentrates on the numbers, the micro, the physical and tangible blood and guts, while the Eastern focuses on the unseen, the macro, the energy, the interplay among our surroundings, thoughts, and feelings. The integration of the two methods of medical practice is essential in finding true health resolutions. With the help of this book, you'll move beyond the nuts and bolts of basic kidney function and learn to look at the kidneys with a new perspective, one that will serve you well in your quest for radiant health.

WHY CLEANSE THE KIDNEYS WHEN THERE ARE SO MANY OTHER CLEANSES?

In my practice working with clients and also in talking with top health practitioners, I have become increasingly aware that starting with kidney cleansing is imperative, no matter the health goal. The kidneys are critical to the body's natural detoxification process and to its innate ability to generate energy on a very primal level. Without proper kidney function, a person is unable to accrue the vigor and willpower needed to overcome health obstacles or properly eliminate harmful substances.

Although both colon cleansing and liver/gallbladder cleansing are also essential, those cleanses move toxins into the bloodstream, which then must be filtered and excreted by the kidneys. If the kidneys are not able to perform effectively, then the toxins re-enter the bloodstream as well as accumulate in the kidneys. This process can lead to inflammation, toxicity, and an increase in symptoms bodywide, defeating the purpose of a cleanse. I believe it is vital to cleanse the kidneys first to open up a detoxification pathway so that all other metabolic processes are properly supported and toxins can be appropriately and effectively removed from the body.

You could compare the cleansing process to clearing a storm drain. If a storm drain is clogged with leaves, branches, and dirt, does it make more sense to push the congested material through by applying high-pressure water from the top or to pull it out from the bottom? If you try to push it through, most likely you will further compress the material, barely getting anything out the bottom, but if you pull it from the bottom, you will relieve the congestion and allow the water to pass through. This is why the kidneys should be cleansed first. In some ways they sit at the "bottom" of the detoxification chain, while the intestines, liver, and gallbladder sit toward the "top." It is vital to clear the path for the movement of toxins by working from the bottom up. Furthermore, by working from the bottom, you are more able to avoid those nasty detoxification side effects, such as headaches, body aches, and fatigue, that are so commonly seen with cleansing programs.

WHY CLEANSE AT ALL?

Cleansing is the process of removing toxins from the body, thus allowing your organs or gland systems to repair and function at optimal levels. Once toxins are removed, your body can use its precious resources for other functions such as energy and hormone production. You could view this process as you do your bank account. You have a certain amount in savings, and every month you plan on using a certain amount for your scheduled expenses. But what happens if you run into added expenses you didn't plan for? If you are a good saver, then you have enough to cover those expenses without depleting your savings—but once those added expenses keep coming, you will reach the point where you have nothing left to give.

This is exactly what happens with toxins and cleansing. Toxins are the added expenses, and cleansing is the accumulation of savings. You always want more savings than expenses to ensure that you never go broke. Once you go broke, disease sets in, making it that much more difficult to recover. The importance of cleansing the body is not only to dig yourself out of debt, but also to start creating a safety net so you keep out of debt. The more you invest in your future, the better the chances that you never risk debt. Get it?

HOW DO I KNOW IF I HAVE TO CLEANSE?

Don't look at cleansing the kidneys as just a treatment or solution to a current symptom—also think of it as a way of creating that safety net. By cleansing the kidneys, you have the ability to prevent illness because you are making a stronger body in which disease cannot thrive. Furthermore, the fewer toxins present, the more efficiently the kidneys are able to do their job. Cleansing is vital to your overall wellness and is your true life insurance.

Although we should all practice the art of kidney cleansing, certain factors make cleansing more pressing for some people than others. The best way to determine if you fall into the category of more urgently needing to cleanse your kidneys is to evaluate your risk factors and health goals. If you fall into multiple risk factors or health goals, then this indicates that you have a higher chance of developing kidney-related disorders and should begin cleansing the kidneys as a preventative tool.

RISK FACTORS

- Exposure to heavy metals (workplace, dental amalgams, tap water)
- Excess aluminum exposure
- Smoking
- History of cystitis and polycystic kidney disease
- History of kidney stones
- Diabetes
- Lupus
- Liver disease
- Sickle cell anemia
- Congestive heart failure
- Chronic high blood pressure (hypertension)
- Use of diuretics (substances that promote urination)
- Diet high in animal protein, sodium, caffeine, fried foods, and refined white sugar
- Soft drink consumption
- Chronic stress
- Living in a hot climate
- Athlete

HEALTH GOALS

- Planning for pregnancy
- Increased energy
- Prevention of kidney disease or kidney stones
- Prevention of kidney stone recurrence
- Healthy hair and nail growth
- Improved condition of ears, bones, bone marrow, and teeth
- Low back pain relief
- Improved fertility/sex drive
- Reduced water weight

IS THIS PARTICULAR CLEANSE RIGHT FOR ME?

This kidney cleanse is extremely gentle and has been designed to work with all body types and health states. The all-natural, food-based cleansing techniques will help your body increase its own detoxification capabilities. This cleanse will not force your body to remove toxins that it is not ready to remove, and it will not overly tax your body. While I always recommend that you talk with your doctor before undergoing any cleanse, this cleanse covers all aspects of toxin removal and organ support to ensure that you have a successful, yet pleasant experience, no matter your current health state.

I believe that everyone should perform a kidney cleanse as part of a general wellness and disease-prevention program, and integrating this cleanse into any lifestyle is extremely manageable. So, if you are eager to feel healthy, this cleanse is for you!

CHAPTER ONE

THE STATE OF TOXICITY

The word "toxin" refers to a substance that has the potential to cause something bad to happen in the body and can sometimes even kill. The most common types of toxins are:

- Xenobiotics, or foreign bodies (viruses, disease-causing bacteria, parasites)
- Biological inhalants (molds, pollens)
- Chemicals (DDT, PCBs, pesticides, herbicides, chlorine)
- Drugs and alcohol
- Heavy metals

When toxins enter the body, they are carried to the liver via the bloodstream and are put in line to be processed. The liver processes toxins through a mechanism called phase I and phase II detoxification. It is through this process that the liver converts the toxins into a form that can be safely excreted. Once converted, these substances are passed out of the liver into the bile in the gallbladder and then excreted by the bowels and kidneys. This process is contingent on a few factors. First, your liver requires high levels of nutrients (vitamins, minerals, and antioxidants) to complete the process, and if not enough of those nutrients are present, then the toxins cannot be processed. Second, if the liver is overburdened by a large toxic load or has been damaged, then it won't be able to process the toxins effectively. Therefore, it is imperative for you to support this process so that these unhealthy substances can be detoxified and made ready for your kidneys to excrete.

The detoxification system assumes that your bile is flowing properly, that your bowels are moving and discharging waste daily, and that your kidneys are properly sorting toxins into your urine and eliminating them. If any of these processes are hindered, then the toxins become stuck in the body. Once toxins have a chance to set up shop in the body, they are either stored in fat tissue (best-case scenario) or they start damaging cells (worst-case scenario). Thus, it is crucial to have the eliminatory, or detoxification, organs functioning properly to get these bad guys out as soon as they come in—which is the ultimate goal of the kidney cleanse.

ARE TOXINS OKAY IN SMALL AMOUNTS?

It depends. If your eliminatory organs are functioning properly and your overall toxic load is low, then yes, you can handle small amounts of toxins. But this is just not the situation for most people. When companies tell you that exposure to small amounts of chemicals in products such shampoo, toothpaste, and perfume is okay, they are not accounting for all the other toxic exposures you encounter on a daily basis. The important thing is not how toxic a single exposure is, but rather your total exposure on a daily basis. Your total toxic load accounts for all your daily exposures—think food, air, and water—and whether you are able to properly process those toxins. It is necessary not only to reduce your exposure, but also to work on repairing your body by increasing the function of your elimination organs, starting with the prime blood cleanser, the kidneys.

THE STATE OF TOXICITY

The first thing to understand is that we are living in an era of constant exposure to toxins at levels never experienced before. We are exposed all day every day through the air we breathe, the food we eat, the water we drink, and the products we use. The human body was not engineered to deal with these high levels of toxins, which means that symptoms of dysfunction are the norm and disease is practically inevitable. While I don't mean to scare you, I want to impress on you the importance of your active participation in your health. The old definition of "healthy"—eating a balanced diet, sleeping eight or more hours a night, and exercising a few times a week—is no longer going to cut it.

As is true for each individual, you are faced with taking a defensive posture on your own health, which requires your vested interest and action. You can't just be a passenger—you are being called to step up and take control. I am going to make this as painless as possible, because regaining control of your health is the most empowering thing you can ever do, providing a level of happiness that you may not have thought possible. I know it's a lofty claim, but I am ready to back it up.

IF TOXINS ARE EVERYWHERE, WHY SHOULD YOU CARE?

You're probably aware that you are exposed to toxins daily—in the forms of gasoline fumes from pumping gas or driving in traffic, toxins from pesticides, second-hand cigarette smoke, or paint and household cleaning products with skull and crossbones on the label—but I am not convinced that you are truly aware of the volume.

There are currently about 75,000 chemicals approved for use in the United States, and about 2,000 more approved each year. The government has tallied 5,000 chemical ingredients in cosmetics, more than 3,200 chemicals added to food, 1,010 chemicals in consumer products, and 500 chemicals used as active ingredients in pesticides. While you won't come into contact with all of these chemicals, you are exposed to more than you might think. This leads to the question I am so often asked: If I am exposed to toxins everywhere, why should I care, especially enough to do a kidney cleanse?

According to a 2004 report in the *British Medical Journal*, "it is clear that environmental and lifestyle factors are key determinants of human disease—accounting for perhaps 75% of most cancers" due to the alarmingly high levels of toxins found in human tissues. Did they say 75%? That alarming percentage helps to explain why diseases and cancers seem to arise out of nowhere, especially when a person appears to be living a relatively healthy life. I don't know about you, but that percentage is high enough to get my attention, and possibly enough to answer the question of why you should care.

When we are exposed to toxins, they often accumulate in our fat tissue, blood, and organs (including the kidneys) and do not necessarily just pass right out the other end. Their passing right through is a misconception that veils the truth of what toxic exposure means and why we should listen up. While the body does have sophisticated detoxification mechanisms, these systems were not intended to take on the volume of toxins they are presented with today. They are unable to properly remove the toxins because of the sheer volume, and they are hindered by our poor nutritional status (yes, even someone who eats vegetables daily can be nutrient deficient) and the progressive breakdown of body systems from daily wear and tear.

What does the body do with the toxins if it can't excrete them? The answer is to store the toxins in much the same way that we stuff, shove, and crowd old belongings and keepsakes we can't part with into the attic, basement, closets, garage, and cubbyholes. Recent estimates show that most Americans have somewhere between 400 and 800 chemicals stored in their bodies at any given time.

To make matters worse, these toxins are found not just in our tissues, but in unborn babies as well. A study by the Environmental Working Group found an average of 200 industrial chemicals and pollutants in umbilical cord blood. These included pesticides, consumer product ingredients, flame retardants, and waste from burning coal, gasoline, and garbage, the majority of which are known to cause cancer. We are exposed to an onslaught of toxins from the beginning of life. Can you imagine that? It would be like a newborn stuck in a crate in grandma's attic surrounded by a hoarder's dream with barely enough room to breathe.

Right now, I am sure you are thinking that those statistics don't apply to you because you're not exposed to toxins all that often. Right? Unfortunately, they apply to all of us. When I said that we were exposed everywhere, I mean everywhere, and the shocking fact is that our exposure comes from places you might never think of. For example, the following are places most people come into contact with daily and the toxins most likely lingering there.

INDOORS: Dust mites; flame retardants (PBDEs) in pillows, mattresses, electronics, drapes, furniture, and carpet; mold and fungus; formaldehyde; VOCs (volatile organic compounds) from paint, carpet, and furniture; phthalates and PVC (polyvinyl chloride) from shower curtains, vinyl floors, and window and wall coverings; lead from paint; pesticides tracked indoors.

FOOD: Antibiotics in nonorganic meat and dairy; dioxins in animal products; herbicides; pesticides; fungicides; phthalates and PVC from plastic wrap and plastic containers; heavy metals (fish); chloroform; perfluorooctanoic acid from nonstick cookware and microwave popcorn; BPA from metal cans, plastic packaging, and coffee makers; MSG; artificial colors and dyes.

TAP WATER: Prescription drugs, birth control pills, chlorine, fluoride, heavy metals, chloroform, perfluorooctanoic acid. (Phthalates and PVC from bottled water.)

COSMETICS: Lead, formaldehyde, triclocarban (bar soap) and triclosan (liquid soap), retinyl palmitate and retinol, fragrance, PEGs (polyethylene glycols), ceteareth-20, parabens, DMDM hydantoin, toluene, DBP (dibutyl phthalate), phthalates, benzalkonium chloride.

CLEANING PRODUCTS: DEA (diethanolamine), TEA (triethanolamine), fragrance, sodium hydroxide, ammonia, chlorine.

OUTDOOR AIR POLLUTION: Benzene (gasoline); perchloroethylene (dry cleaners); methylene chloride (solvent and paint stripper); dioxin; asbestos; toluene; formaldehyde; and metals such as cadmium, mercury, chromium, and lead compounds.

Okay, okay, so I have not exactly answered the question of why, if toxins are everywhere, you should care enough to do something about protecting yourself—like performing a kidney cleanse.

The way I see it, each person has a different motive, a different trigger. For me, I care because I want to live a healthy life—free of pain, full of energy and vitality, still with it, moving and shaking at age 100, able to see my great grandkids climbing all over me. For you, this may not be your dream, so choose one of these other reasons to care:

- I don't want to get cancer or another serious or terminal illness.
- I have a family history of disease, putting me at high risk, and I don't want to succumb to history.
- I currently have a disease and am looking for options to bring myself out of it.

- I plan to get pregnant and want to be as fertile as possible, and I don't want my baby to have toxins in the umbilical cord.
- I'm tired and I'm tired of being tired.
- My looks are important to me, and since the health of my insides dictates the beauty of my outsides, I want to be as healthy and beautiful as possible.
- I am exhibiting symptoms of kidney problems and am motivated to stop them.
- I am a parent and want to live as long as possible and see my children grow up.
- I love the feeling of being healthy and want to see how great I can actually feel.
- Health, including cleansing, is a hobby, and this is a new avenue for me to explore.
- I know my toxin levels are high, and I have a sneaking suspicion that they are leading to some of my aches and pains.
- I am dealing with some weird symptoms that no one has been able to figure out, and cleansing seems like the road to salvation.
- I am detecting signs of aging, such as wrinkles and cellulite, and freeing myself of toxins is the path to the fountain of youth.

Whatever your reason, I commend you and can assure you that you are in for a fabulous ride. Although there may be a few rain showers and thunderstorms along the way, the destination is worth the trouble!

Now that we are crystal clear on toxins and how pervasive they are, let's talk about how to eliminate them through detoxification.

"Detoxification" is another word for "cleansing"—the physiological or medicinal removal of toxic substances from the body. We have all thrown these terms around, but I would guess that not many people actually know what they mean. We know that we must cleanse to offset our bad behaviors such as drinking alcohol, eating junk food, and smoking, but what is actually happening inside the body that makes this process so important?

Our bodies detoxify naturally every day by eliminating or neutralizing toxins through the colon, liver, lungs, kidneys, lymphatic system, and skin. It is a necessary metabolic function because the body continually accumulates toxins from both internal and external sources. For example, did you know that the very process of breathing is a form of detoxification? Carbon dioxide is a naturally occurring toxin in the body that is removed or detoxified via the lungs through exhalation. This is just one of many ways in which the body creates toxins through metabolic processes and then removes them.

The problem is that while the body was engineered to clear these naturally occurring toxins, it faces new challenges when more and more external toxins are added to the overall load. Remember the term "toxic load"? The question becomes, how can we promote the removal of both internally generated and external toxins?

The main goal of detoxifying or cleansing the body is to reduce exposure to, minimize the internal creation of, and promote the clearance of toxins. To reduce exposure, you will be modifying your diet and your lifestyle habits and moving toward toxin-free products. To minimize the internal creation of toxins, you will be improving the way in which you metabolize. Finally, to promote the clearance of toxins, you will be using practices that support the movement of toxins out of your tissues. These practices involve methods such as fasting, diet modification, and targeted nutrition, in addition to therapies such as saunas, castor oil packs, yoga, and dry brushing.

HEAVY METALS AND CHEMICALS

The following is a list of heavy metals and chemicals that have been shown to harm the kidneys and where they are often found. Please use this list as a guide to reduce or eliminate your exposure.

MERCURY

- Dental amalgams
- Seafood (shark, tuna, swordfish, tilefish)
- Fungicides used on lawns and often on grains
- Air contamination from coal burning and the incineration
- of mercury-containing equipment
- Air conditioner filters
- Tattoos
- Thermometers
- Light bulbs (high-intensity discharge, florescent)

- Personal care products: Skin-lightening creams, antiseptic creams and ointments (for psoriasis), body powders, cosmetics, suppositories

ARSENIC

- Apple juice
- Rice products
- Drinking water, well water, groundwater
- Baby food, processed and infant rice cereals
- Seafood (shellfish)
- Wine
- Tobacco
- Rat poisons
- Wood preservatives
- Fertilizers, feed additives, insecticides, pesticides
- Industrial processing (glass, paper, textiles, pigments)

LEAD

- Car exhaust
- Canned foods
- Hair dyes
- Tap water (from lead pipes and tanks)
- Newsprint
- Lead house paint
- Rainwater
- Pencils
- Cosmetics (lipstick)
- Pottery glaze
- Cigarette smoke

CADMIUM

- Evaporated milk
- Shellfish (especially oysters)
- Refined foods (especially refined wheat flour)
- Organ meat
- Tap water (especially soft water from galvanized pipes)
- Soft drinks
- Sewage sludge
- Paint
- Cigarette smoke
- Fungicides, fertilizers

URANIUM

- Air pollution (uranium mines, coal-fired power plants, nuclear power plants)
- Tap water, well water
- Root vegetables
- Ceramic and porcelain glaze
- X-rays

COPPER

- Copper electrical wiring
- Copper cooking utensils and cookware
- Building materials containing copper
- Fungicides, algicides, insecticides
- Wood preservatives
- Animal feeds
- Food additives (coloring agents)
- Tap water (from copper pipes)

BISMUTH

- Fishing anchors
- Shotgun pellets
- Cosmetics
- Pharmaceuticals
- Soldering fumes

CHEMICALS TO AVOID IN PERSONAL CARE PRODUCTS

- Parabens
- DEA (diethanolamine), TEA (triethanolamine)
- Sodium lauryl/laureth sulfate
- Petroleum/petroleum jelly
- PPG (propylene glycol), PEG (polyethylene glycol), polyoxyethylene, polyethoxyethylene, polyethoxyethylene mineral oil
- Fragrance/parfum
- Synthetic colors and dyes (blue 1, green 3, yellow 5 and 6, red 33)
- Aluminum
- Phthalates
- 1,4-dioxine
- Petrolatum
- Lead acetate
- Triclosan, chloro, phenol, irgasan
- Isobutene

CHEMICALS TO AVOID IN HOUSEHOLD CLEANING PRODUCTS

- Sodium hypochlorate, sodium hydroxide
- Ammonia
- Phenol, cresol
- Nitrobenzene, para-dichlorobenzene
- Phosphates
- Perchloroethylene, diethylene glycol
- Petroleum distillates/ solvents
- Naphthalene
- Dioxins
- Chlorinated phenols
- Nonylphenol ethoxylate
- Formaldehyde
- Butyl cellosolve
- Triclosan
- Quarternary ammonium compounds, or QUATS (antibacterial)
- 2-butoxyethanol

CHAPTER TWO

THE KIDNEYS AND THEIR ROLE IN HEALTH

Knowledge is the key to making a true change in your health. It is just as important to understand why you are doing something as it is to do it. Instead of jumping right into cleansing, start with a basic understanding of the role of kidneys. If you respect the kidneys for all they do in the body, you'll want to treat them the way they deserve to be treated. And don't worry, if you just cringed at the thought of an anatomy lesson, this will be short and sweet.

THE KIDNEYS AND HOW THEY WORK

The kidneys remove waste and water from the blood, and they form urine, one of the body's main ways to rid itself of toxins. But how does waste get into the blood in the first place? It gets into the blood through the normal metabolism of active tissues, such as muscles, as well as from components of foods we eat, such as sugars, food coloring, preservatives, and MSG. It is important to note that we are using our food as fuel, and so any components that are not good for us are sent directly to the blood as waste. The more junk you eat, the more waste you are forcing your body to deal with. Get it?

If the kidneys are unable to remove this waste, then it builds back up in the blood and damages the body, including the kidneys. It is crucial that our kidneys perform their role efficiently, because just as you do not want to live in a house full of waste, neither do your cells.

How exactly do the kidneys remove the waste? The actual process of waste removal occurs inside tiny units in the kidneys called nephrons. Each kidney contains millions of nephrons housing intricate filtering and balancing systems. Once the waste enters a nephron, it goes into a tiny blood vessel called a glomerulus that intertwines with a urine-collecting tube called a tubule. The glomerulus filters the waste out of the blood, into a collecting duct, and out of the kidney via the ureter to be eliminated through urination.

During this process of filtering waste, many other vital functions are happening as well. Let's take a quick look at them.

URINE FORMATION AND BLOOD CLEANSING

Through the formation of urine, the kidneys act as one of the most important detoxification organs in the body, expelling about 1½ liters of urine each day. It is one of the most efficient ways for the body to rid itself of toxins and impurities that could otherwise damage the blood and lead to bodywide dysfunction.

The formation of urine involves filtration, reabsorption, and secretion. To remember this process, think of FRS (or my mnemonic, first-rate secretor). This is where the body chooses the nutrients it needs to keep and what it must get rid of.

FILTRATION: The kidneys receive about 200 liters of blood a day for filtration. Wait, let's think about how much that is. A medium carton of milk holds about 1 liter (equal to about a quart), so imagine having to filter 200 quart-size containers of blood a day! And, remember, each kidney is only the size of a computer mouse.

REABSORPTION: Water, sugars, amino acids, vitamins, toxins, and other substances are processed from this enormous load of blood volume. They are either filtered into urine or reabsorbed back into the blood. If it's good and needed, like important minerals such as calcium, then it's filtered back into the blood system for use. We don't want to throw out valuables, do we? About 99% of substances are reabsorbed, leaving only about 1½ liters of urine to be excreted.

SECRETION: Toxic waste products such as hydrogen ions, potassium ions, and drugs are secreted into the urine for excretion. Remember how we talked about the toxins from the food we eat? Well, those guys are being addressed here. Sayonara, see ya later!

Once urine is formed, it is sent down a long tube called the ureter to the urinary bladder, a sac that holds the urine. Once the bladder starts to fill up, your body gets the message that you have to pee. When you pee, the urine travels from the urinary bladder through the urethra, a duct that carries the urine out of the body.

Now, hold on tight as we look at how, through the FRS process, the kidneys control six functions that are vital for our health and wellness.

1. PH (ACID-ALKALINE) BALANCE

Your blood's pH—also referred to as your acid-alkaline balance—is one of the most telling signs of health. pH, which stands for "the potential of hydrogen" is measured on a scale of 0 to 14. The neutral point is 7.0. pH levels below 7 are progressively more acidic, and above 7 are progressively more alkaline. pH is a vital marker of health, and a very slight deviation can greatly influence body functions.

The kidneys help to maintain blood plasma at pH 7.4. By regulating pH, the kidneys help to maintain a healthy environment, which promotes the efficient function of all biosystems.

This vital organ pair plays a primary role in maintaining pH balance by selecting which ions to retain and which ones to excrete. This allows the body's total acid burden to be constant, as the urine's acidity fluctuates to accommodate the balance. If the blood is too acidic, meaning that there is an excess of hydrogen ions, the kidneys move these ions to the urine for excretion as a means of alkalizing the blood. If the blood is too alkaline, meaning there is a deficiency of hydrogen ions, the kidneys hold onto these ions to acidify the blood. In a healthy body, pH is managed and kept in balance at all times.

2. BLOOD VOLUME AND PRESSURE

The kidneys are a vital component in maintaining healthy blood volume and blood pressure. Based on the level of blood volume and the amount of blood that circulates through the kidneys, the kidneys determine how much water you need to excrete as well as hold onto. If blood pressure is too low, the kidneys hold onto water. If blood pressure is too high, the kidneys allow for more water to be passed through urination.

The kidneys receive 25% of the blood that exits the heart, and it is the kidneys' job to monitor that blood flow to control pressure. The kidneys meticulously adjust the volume and concentration of urine to accommodate changes in the body, including variations in daily food and beverage intake. Various hormones, proteins, and enzymes found in the body—antidiuretic hormone (ADH), renin, angiotensin, and aldosterone—come into play in the adjustments the kidneys make on whether to retain or release water or dissolved substances.

3. FLUID AND ELECTROLYTE (SODIUM) BALANCE

The kidneys control the body's water content through the water-retaining hormone ADH. When ADH is present, the body decreases the amount of urine formed and less water is lost. When ADH is not present, the amount of urine formed increases and more water is lost. This is a very delicate balancing act.

The control of electrolytes is monitored through aldosterone, a sodium- and water-retaining hormone. When sodium is low, aldosterone stimulates the kidneys to reabsorb sodium, increasing water reabsorption and decreasing water lost from urine. Therefore, any dysfunction in the kidneys can cause symptoms such as water retention, also known as edema.

4. WASTE EXCRETION

The main function of the kidneys is to excrete toxins and waste products that accumulate in the blood, thereby cleansing the blood. Some of the main toxins that the kidneys cleanse are nitrogenous waste products, such as ammonia and urea, resulting from the breakdown of proteins. If the kidneys are not functioning properly, often because of high intake of animal protein (meat, poultry, fish, eggs, and dairy products), their ability to filter out these toxins is greatly reduced, which can lead to problems such as gout and kidney stones.

5. HORMONE SECRETIONS AND RED BLOOD CELL PRODUCTION

Red blood cells are oxygen carriers. Without oxygen in our cells, we die, so red blood cell levels must be maintained at all times. The kidneys have an important role in this job. When oxygen levels are low, the kidneys get the message to secrete a hormone called erythropoietin, which signals the bone marrow to increase production of red blood cells until oxygen levels are normalized. Pretty slick, huh?

6. VITAMIN D UTILIZATION AND BONE HEALTH

Vitamin D has finally been recognized for its amazing benefits, including cold and flu prevention, bone health, inflammation reduction, and the inhibition of cancer cells. But you probably didn't know that the kidneys play a role in vitamin D use in the body.

When the body comes into contact with sunlight, UVB wavelengths react with 7-dehydrocholesterol, a cholesterol precursor. This reaction forms Vitamin D3. In order for it to be utilized as vitamin D, it must go through two reactions, one in the liver and one in the kidneys. Thus, in order to maintain healthy vitamin D levels in the body, you have to have functioning kidneys.

Now that we have a clear understanding of the kidneys' role in the body from a Western perspective, I want to take a moment to look at their role from an Eastern perspective, specifically traditional Chinese medicine. This is where the true magic lies. Chinese medicine teaches us that the kidneys are in control of so many more functions than are known in the West. Viewing kidney health and disease from both perspectives results in a broader, more comprehensive approach to cleansing and far more effective results.

THE KIDNEYS: THE ROOT OF LIFE

In Chinese medicine, the kidneys—known as the root of life, gate of life, minister of power, and home of the heaven constitution—are of prime importance to the body. These epithets reveal how the kidneys' roles go far beyond urine generation and waste excretion. While Western medicine limits its description and understanding of the kidneys to the actual organ, traditional Chinese medicine assigns a more profound and broad significance to them. Chinese medicine believes that our kidneys are our very foundation, the most deep-seated of all of the organs and encompassing not just the kidneys themselves but also the adrenal glands. This connection is vital to understanding the perspective of Chinese medicine, because you cannot talk about the kidney without also referring to the adrenal glands. They are one and the same conceptually, and so any reference to the word "kidneys" in Chinese medicine includes the adrenal glands.

So why are the kidneys referred to as the root of life? The kidneys are the root or rather the home of the *jing*, the original qi (chi), which constitutes our very life force. It is this life force that is responsible for providing the foundation and tools required to fulfill our deepest human needs: survival and reproduction, life and death. The kidneys:

- Store the *jing*, the inherited constitution
- Receive the qi, or energy
- Control the gate of life/*ming men* (minister fire)

In Chinese medicine, the kidneys are viewed in relationship to the systems with which they interact: the bladder, the endocrine system, and especially the adrenal glands. The kidneys are seen as containing vital energies that have influence over the meridians, or energy pathways, to which all body functions are intimately tied. This philosophy is what we refer to as holistic, meaning that each and every system of the body has influence over another—and in this case, the kidneys are the foundation. The kidneys influence not just physical processes such as mineral balance and waste excretion, but also emotional processes such as feelings of fear and anxiety because the kidneys house the *jing*.

Without losing you completely in the mysteries of Chinese medicine, I will share with you a little knowledge about how this ancient medicine provides vital tools with which to view and understand the kidneys and their key to whole body revitalization and radiant health.

JING: THE ESSENCE

The kidneys store the *jing*, or life essence, the deepest source of energy, our inherited potential for life, that which determines our ability to survive and reproduce.

GROWTH, DEVELOPMENT, AND REPRODUCTION

Jing, specifically prenatal *jing*, is largely responsible for our growth and development, mental and physical power, and our ability to reproduce. It is the electrical force from which our sexual life is derived—the energy that grows out of the sperm and egg. For example, conception is made possible by the inherited power of *jing*, growth to maturity is the blossoming of *jing*, and aging reflects the weakening of *jing*. It is the deepest source of energy in the body and is associated with genetics. *Jing* is also our long-term energy and may be thought of as our reserves of life force, although I like to think of it as our gusto. The preservation of the *jing* is key to longevity and health.

These are the characteristics attributed to *jing*:

- Longevity
- Youthfulness
- Vitality
- Mental energy/acuity
- Reproductive power
- Regeneration

BONE MARROW, BONES, BRAIN, TEETH, AND HAIR

Kidney *jing* is also in charge of the production of bone marrow, which is viewed as being able to generate the spinal cord and "fill up" the brain, thereby providing us with memory, mental acuity, and creative force. Because bone marrow also ensures strong bones and teeth, addressing the *jing* is critical when dealing with conditions related to the bones and teeth.

In addition to driving the production of bone marrow, kidney *jing* also drives the spinal marrow, a vital part of mental development and brain function as well as hair growth. When kidney *jing* is strong, head hair is abundant and its growth strong. And when kidney *jing* is depleted or weak, hair loses its color and falls out.

For a long time I dealt with hair loss and went the conventional route of supplementing with basic vitamins such as biotin, zinc, and B vitamins, but without success. Then I was introduced to a Chinese tonic herbal formula designed to target kidney *jing*. My hair grew back thicker and longer. The results were and continue to be astounding. As a result of nourishing the kidneys and consequently the *jing*, my hair has never been healthier. This product quickly became part of my nutrition practice and has provided similar results to others. I know I sound like an infomercial, but the connections are extremely strong. By strengthening kidney *jing*, you increase the chi, which rises to the head hair, resulting in healthy hair. In my practice, targeting the kidneys has proved to be the most effective way to increase hair growth and strengthen the hair follicles. Nothing like real-life proof!

PRESERVING *JING*

Jing is often referred to as prenatal *jing*, because it is inherited in a fixed amount at birth. The amount we are born with is the amount we have to spend throughout our lifetime, so often it is referred to as our *jing* reserve. The more *jing*, the better we are able to maintain our health and youthfulness and promote longevity. Therefore, the goal is to prolong the essence by not dipping into those reserves and by engaging in activities that reduce its depletion. We are going to do this during the cleanse not only by eliminating *jing*-depleting activities, but also by consuming adaptogenic herbs. These specialized herbs are of vital importance to the cleanse because they minimize *jing* depletion, thus promoting radiant health. The kidneys are the storehouse of the richest and most concentrated ancestral energy, inherited and passed through generations.

What Are Adaptogenic Herbs?

Adaptogenic herbs are specialized tonic herbs that enhance the mind and body's capacity to adapt to and endure life's stressors and changes. By supporting the body, they increase physical, mental, and emotional fortitude. Essentially, these herbs provide resilience, so that you do not have to tap into your deeper life essence (*jing*) or reserves to overcome stress. Think of the herbs as building your body armor or providing you with super powers. The adaptogenic herbs astragalus and *Cordyceps sinensis* are the tools you will use to minimize your depletion of *jing* while on the kidney cleanse.

DEPLETION OF *JING*

Unfortunately, our kidney *jing* reserves are delicate and can easily become depleted, which emphasizes the importance of supporting the kidneys with adaptogenic herbs while cleansing. *Jing* energy is depleted by the act of living, and we have no control over that, but it can also be rapidly depleted by external stressors. Some of these stressors are anxiety, fear, poor nutrition, and toxic buildup in the kidneys. The goal is to eliminate as many external stressors as possible during the cleanse.

When the *jing* is depleted, premature aging occurs, leading not only to early onset of gray hair, but also to reproductive and developmental disorders and a shortened lifespan. By cleansing the kidneys (and consuming adaptogenic herbs during the cleanse), we are able to preserve our *jing* and thus our inherited life force, delay the aging process, and push back the classic signs of depleted *jing*.

As the ancient texts of Chinese medicine say, *So hair and beard go white, the body grows heavy, the step is not so sure, one no Longer Has Children.*

THE KIDNEYS: UNDERSTANDING THE YIN AND YANG

Now that we have covered the philosophy of *jing*, let's take a look at the other guiding principle of traditional Chinese medicine: yin and yang. Yin and yang are opposite forces that are constantly in motion, creating an everchanging balance in the body. While opposing, they create an integrated whole with one force always trying to dominate the other. No dominance is permanent, hence their creation of a stable whole. The rhythmic nature of these opposing forces is what establishes the basis of all things, including health.

Yin is characterized as the essential life force: cold, moist, damp, and relaxing. Yang is seen as the creator: hot, dry, mobile, and invigorating. Yin is where energy is accumulated, and yang where the energy is expended. It is by finding this dynamic yet harmonious balance that radiant health is achieved.

Yin's physiological aspects

- Cooling
- Reduced metabolism (hypometabolic)
- Receptive
- Building (anabolic)
- Maintaining

Deficiency of yin (excess of yang—hypermetabolic)

- Nervousness
- Anxiety
- Insomnia
- Dryness
- Flushness
- Inflammation

Yang's physiological aspects

- Warming
- Increased metabolism (hypermetabolic)
- Aggressive
- Breaking down (catabolic)
- Protective

Deficiency of yang (excess of yin—hypometabolic)

- Fatigue
- Weakness
- Low vitality
- Edema
- Paleness
- Coldness

In Chinese medicine, kidney *jing* is differentiated into either yin or yang.

In the kidneys, the left kidney is yin, the water element, while the right kidney is yang, the fire element. Our entire being relies on the constant balance of these two qualities, the building up and breaking down of nutrients and tissues (the anabolic and catabolic processes). When kidney yin and yang are balanced, the yin and yang of the other organs in the body are also stabilized. Conversely, when kidney yin and yang are out of balance, the body's other organs follow suit.

Kidney Yin

Kidney yin is related to the parasympathetic ("rest and digest") nervous system and the hormone cortisol, which is released from the adrenal cortex. It is responsible for restoration and revitalization—the key to core vitality. This includes protein, carbohydrate and fat metabolism, and inflammation and stress responses. If the body is under prolonged stress, yin deficiency can occur, leading to a state where the body cannot repair nor maintain itself.

As Daverick Leggett, author of *Recipes for Self-Healing*, says, "Yin is like a well which must not run dry, a reserve of nutrients which form the basis of growth and the fuel for all physiological activities."

The following are common signs of kidney yin deficiencies (meaning the adrenals are fatigued):

- Dizziness
- Constipation
- Hot flashes
- Insomnia
- Anxiety
- Vertigo
- Sore back

Kidney Yang

Kidney yang is related to the sympathetic ("fight or flight") nervous system and to the hormones, norepinepherine and epinephrine, which are released from the adrenal medulla. When yin and yang go out of balance and yang deficiency occurs, symptoms such as weakness, tinnitus, pain in the lumbar region, vertigo, mental confusion, and problems with the sex organs arise. Therefore, it is of prime importance to have a constant balance between the yin and yang so that neither becomes deficient.

The following are common signs of kidney yang deficiencies:

- Aversion to cold
- Fatigue
- Poor appetite
- Fertility issues
- Edema
- Adrenal fatigue
- Weak lower limbs

THE GOVERNOR OF WATER

In Chinese medicine organs are attributed to an element, and it is only fitting that the kidney belongs to the element of water. Much as in Western medicine, one of the prime roles of the kidneys in Chinese medicine is to regulate the distribution, regulation, and excretion of water. The kidneys contribute to the excretion of waste products while maintaining a proper pH through their ability to balance minerals, but these processes are believed to rely on the warming and pushing function of kidney yang.

THE KIDNEYS AND HEARING

When you think of conditions such as hearing loss and tinnitus, you probably do not look to the kidneys, but Chinese medicine offers a different perspective. When you have an issue with the ears, you don't address the ears directly, but rather the kidneys. *The Yellow Emperor's Classic of Internal Medicine*, a traditional Chinese medicine text, states, "The kidney's chi [energy] goes through the ear. If the kidney is harmonized, the ear can hear the five tones." The interesting thing is that while Western medicine doesn't connect deficiencies or conditions of the ear to the kidney and vice versa, the medical community does recognize several areas of similarities between the ears and kidneys such as their structure, function, and the timing of prenatal development.

Another aspect of the relationship between the kidneys and the ears is the role of uric acid and mineral crystals. When the kidneys are unable to filter properly because of excessive buildup of waste products in the form of uric acid and minerals, these waste products form into crystals. Traditional Chinese medical practitioners believe that the crystals are deposited in various parts of the body such as the joints and the inner ear, which can lead to issues with hearing. As a result, the ability of the kidney to filter and to clear crystal deposits is critical to ear health.

THE KIDNEYS AND WILLPOWER

The kidneys are related to emotional processes as well as physical functions. Kidney qi is also referred to as willpower. "The Kidneys determine our will power," according to Giovanni Maciocia, author of *The Foundations of Chinese Medicine*. "If the Kidneys are strong, the will power will be strong, the mind will be focused on goals that it sets itself and it will pursue them in a single-minded way. Conversely, if the Kidneys are weak, will power will be lacking and the mind will be easily discouraged and swayed from its aims."

PUTTING IT ALL TOGETHER

It is through the perspective of traditional Chinese medicine that we can truly see the far-reaching effects of the kidneys. By addressing the kidneys, we can tap into the life force of the body, which controls far more than pH, fluid balance, and waste excretion. We are taking a lesson from Eastern practitioners and recognizing the importance of cleansing the kidneys and supporting the cleanse with adaptogenic herbs.

These are the main characteristics of the kidneys in Chinese medicine:

- Peak energy hours 5 to 7 a.m.
- Govern birth, growth, reproduction, development, sexual vitality, aging
- Control willpower, express ambition and focus
- Control bones, particularly lumbar spine and knees
- Produce marrow
- Nourish brain to sustain concentration, clear thinking, skill ability, memory
- Facilitate inspiration
- Control teeth, head hair, ears (hearing), equilibrium
- Emotional expression of feeling grounded, feeling courageous, having willpower and endurance

The following are signs of kidney deficiency or dysfunction:

- Indecisiveness, fear in pit of stomach
- Cold feet and legs
- Abundant swelling, edema
- Bladder issues
- Fearfulness, anxiety, insecurity, antisocial tendencies
- Chronic fatigue
- Lack of will, impatience, discouragement, laziness
- Low sex drive
- Sciatica, lumbago
- Inflammation, musculoskeletal irritation
- Dreams (when kidneys are weak) of drowning, swimming after a shipwreck; of being immersed in water; as if the back and waist are split apart, spine is detached from body

CHAPTER THREE

SIGNS OF TOXIC KIDNEYS

Did you know that the majority of us are dealing with some sort of kidney dysfunction?

Yes, that's correct, but we are not trained to recognize the symptoms. We are conditioned to the Western model of medicine, meaning that we are told the symptom or problem we are facing is due to a diagnosable condition or is simply "normal"—but there is a large gray area in between the two responses. It is precisely that gray area I want shed light on because that's where cleansing practices and preventive medicine can make a huge difference.

When I refer to a gray area, I mean when an organ or gland system is no longer functioning at optimal level but has yet to reach a point where it can be diagnosed as a condition or disease. You may have ailments and symptoms, but from a Western perspective there is no clear solution for how to deal with them because there is no diagnosis. Your choices are to take a pharmaceutical drug or wait and see what happens.

It's easy to relate to this scenario, as most of us self-medicate for symptoms we are conditioned to view as "normal." These include insomnia, fatigue, headaches, bloating, indigestion, hair loss, dry skin, and constipation. These symptoms are actually messages from our body telling us that something is not right, an organ or gland system is not functioning properly, and the longer we ignore these symptoms or continue to self-medicate, the greater the chances that the symptoms will turn into a real diagnosable condition.

Therefore, to really see the signs of a toxic kidney, you must begin to look at "normal" symptoms that often lie in the gray area and recognize that they may be warning signs of kidney toxicity and aren't "normal" after all. Once you are able to identify these signs, you can then see the value in the kidney cleanse as a tool to increase kidney function—which in turn leads to symptom relief as well as prevention of any impending disease or condition.

IDENTIFYING THE SYMPTOMS OF KIDNEY TOXICITY

Kidney disease? Kidney stones? Dialysis? Even if any of you are not dealing with a specific kidney condition, please know that this cleanse is still for you. Kidney dysfunction shows up in many ways, the majority of which do not even seem kidney related. But with the incorporation of both Eastern and Western medical practices, we can learn the various ways in which our body tells us our kidneys are hurting. Take a look at the list below, and if you can say yes to any of the following, then you will want to start giving your kidneys some love. I know I did!

- Kidney stones
- Bladder issues/stones
- Chronic urinary tract infections
- Poor bone health
- Poor lymphatic flow/drainage (edema, weak immune system, cellulite, swollen glands, puffiness, allergies)
- Conditions of the bone marrow (anemia, lymphoma, leukemia)
- Loss of hearing or ringing in the ears (tinnitus)
- Dark brown or black circles and/or puffiness under the eyes
- Lack of power and drive
- Social anxiety, ADD, ADHD
- Low sex drive
- Infertility
- Thin skin
- Weak nails
- Foggy head
- Low back pain
- Low energy
- Edema, excess water weight

- Terrible balance, clumsiness
- Feelings of fear
- Poor physical development
- Thinning hair, early onset of gray or white hair
- Menstrual complications

These symptoms indicate less-than-optimal kidney function, but what about potential risk factors that increase your chances of developing kidney problems in the future? The truth is that certain diseases, family histories, diets, and even where you live can contribute to your risk. While your kidneys may not yet be signaling to you that something is wrong, I still encourage you to use this cleanse to protect them and prevent problems from actually manifesting. Take control of your future and your health rather than waiting for nature to take its toll. What do you think about that? Want to keep your kidneys healthy and happy indefinitely? (Say yes!)

Risk factors for kidney dysfunction or disease:

- Adrenal fatigue
- Age: The kidneys begin to get smaller at about age 35 to 40. After you reach 40 years old, the nephrons decrease by 10% every 10 years.
- Alcoholism
- Apple-shaped body: Newer research shows that higher waist-to-hip ratios are associated with lower kidney function, lower kidney blood flow, and higher blood pressure within the kidneys, increasing your risk for kidney disease.
- Chemical exposure (see "Resources" on page 207 for more information)
- Chronic emotional state of fear
- Cigarette smoking
- Frequent bladder infections
- Gender: Men have a higher risk of developing kidney disease.
- Heart disease
- Heavy metal toxicity
- High blood pressure (hypertension) or family history of it
- High cholesterol

- Hyperinsulinemia (excess levels of insulin in the blood)
- Hypoparathyroidism or hyperparathyroid (concentration of parathyroid hormone in the blood)
- Insulin-dependent diabetes or family history of it
- Metabolic syndrome
- Pharmaceutical drug use
- Polycystic kidney disease
- Race and ethnicity: African Americans, Hispanics, Native Americans, and Asians have the highest rates of kidney disease. Caucasians have a lower rate.
- Urinary tract infections
- Vitamin D toxicity

RISK FACTORS FOR KIDNEY STONES (NEPHROLITHIASIS)

- Abnormal testosterone levels
- Acidosis (excess acidity of body fluids or tissues)
- Certain medical conditions: Renal tubular acidosis, cystinuria, urinary tract infections, leukemia, lymphoma, sarcoidosis
- Certain pharmaceutical drugs, especially decongestants, diuretics, protease inhibitors, and anticonvulsants
- Diet: High sodium, high animal protein (and some protein powders), low fiber, low minerals, high caffeine intake, generally poor nutrition
- Digestive diseases including inflammatory bowel disease
- Family history
- Gender: Men are more likely than women to get kidney stones, but that statistic is changing.
- Gout
- High blood pressure (hypertension)
- High stress
- Hyperparathyroidism
- Infection (nanobacteria)
- Insulin resistance

- Kidney deformities
- Living in a warmer climate
- Low urine volume (commonly due to dehydration)
- Obesity
- Poor gut flora
- Surgical menopause
- Vitamin A deficiency

If you have had a kidney stone, then it is very important for you to reduce the risk of recurrence. A prior kidney stone increases your chances of recurrence by 50%, and it also increases your risk of chronic kidney disease, which in turn can increase your risk of a heart attack. Researchers have found that kidney stones increase the risk for a heart attack by more than a third, independent of their effect on chronic kidney disease.

If these lists are not enough to fuel your fire, I don't know what will! It would be sheer luck if you didn't hit at least one of the risk factors, but the positive news is that you can do something about it! If you were not already persuaded to cleanse your kidneys, I really hope you are feeling the conviction now, because it is always much easier to prevent disease and dysfunction rather than to pull yourself out of it (and, in some cases, you can't pull yourself out). You can choose to flow downstream, merely dodging a few rocks, rather than face the struggle of swimming upstream in a torrential storm with rapids. *Capeesh?*

CHAPTER FOUR

PREPARING FOR THE KIDNEY CLEANSE

Before I get into the details of what to do on the cleanse, I want to give you a snapshot of what the kidney cleanse entails. This is the structure you will be following for the next 30 days:

- 4 days of cleanse preparation with gradual dietary modifications
- 3-day juice feast with kidney-specific nutrients and foods
- 3 weeks on the kidney cleanse food plan plus adjunct alternative therapies

I created this kidney cleanse by following the fundamental rules of detoxification taken from both Eastern and Western medical practices. Using knowledge from Western medicine, the cleanse focuses on dietary intake of foods and herbs that increase kidney function while eliminating any substance that can harm the kidneys. And using knowledge from Eastern medicine, the cleanse addresses not just the kidneys, but also their relationship to the body as a whole, the environment, and any disharmony between the two.

Since the various parts of the body are intimately connected, any dysfunction in an organ or gland system impacts and disrupts the overall function of the body. It is impossible to truly cleanse any one organ or gland, especially a detoxifying organ such as the kidneys, without addressing the whole organism. That is what makes this kidney cleanse unique—it cleanses the kidneys while helping to support the cleansing of the system in its entirety. Talk about bang for the buck!

My strategy is to follow the rapid and powerful detoxification effects of a juice cleanse with a nutritional food cleanse to promote the release of deep-rooted toxins while at the same time building kidney strength and function.

You can easily do this cleanse at home as long as you are a willing participant. That means that you will have to make a promise to yourself to dedicate the next month to revitalizing your health. The majority of us dedicate barely 10 minutes a day to ourselves, so the concept of a month may seem staggering, but the point is that you picked up this book for a reason, and you deserve to invest in yourself and especially in your health.

DETOXIFICATION BASICS

REDUCE THE WORKLOAD OF THE DIGESTIVE SYSTEM: Eliminate potential food allergens, toxins, and hard-to-digest foods. This way you are reducing the overall toxic load on your body from both external sources and internal processes (metabolism and poor digestion).

INCREASE CELLULAR ENERGY: Incorporate more liquid-based, raw, and lightly cooked meals to increase available nutrition to cells. This allows cells to more effectively get rid of toxins.

PROVIDE THE TOOLS FOR DETOXIFICATION: Use targeted nutrition, therapeutic herbs, and adjunct therapies to make toxin removal easier for your body.

INCREASE WATER INTAKE: Water serves as a solvent for the removal of toxins. It literally flushes the toxins out!

SUPPORT THE KIDNEYS: The targeted nutrients in the recommended foods, teas, and supplements will increase kidney function and support tissue repair.

SUPPORT BOWEL ELIMINATION: To reduce the toxic load, make sure of proper bowel movements through nutrition, water intake, and adjunct therapies.

HOW THE KIDNEY CLEANSE WILL IMPACT YOUR HEALTH

Although everyone is different, and each of us is on a unique health path, performing this kidney cleanse will most certainly affect your health positively. By eliminating toxic foods and substances, in combination with beneficial healing foods and nutrients, as well as exercises and stress-reduction techniques, you will be giving your body the chance to make profound changes. And these are changes that you can continue to build on after finishing the actual cleanse. While I will do my part to guide you and provide the tools you need, ultimately success is up to you. If you pull your weight and hold up your end, then I can hold up mine, and together we will get you to the point where you begin to see changes.

To give you an idea of what to expect, here is a brief review of changes that may occur both internally and externally:

- Cleansing of old stagnant waste products and bad bacteria from the digestive tract, leading to improved digestion and normal bowel movements
- Reduction in cravings for sugar, caffeine, alcohol, and carbohydrates
- Increased function of the lymphatic and immune systems
- Clearance of excess mucus and congestion
- Improved detoxification ability of the liver
- Clearance of toxic matter, especially from fat tissue, which can lead to weight loss
- Alkaline urinary pH, which promotes an environment that reduces bacteria, virus, fungus, parasites, and disease from flourishing
- Reduction in inflammation, allergies, skin problems, headaches, fatigue, insomnia, and depression
- Alleviation of puffy eyes or dark circles under the eyes
- Improved blood chemistry
- Improved mineral status and thus bone health
- Alleviation of lower back pain
- Healthy hair and nail growth
- Improved sex drive and fertility
- Enhanced mental clarity
- Improved physical performance and drive
- Energy!
- Reduction in water weight, bloating, and edema

- Improvement in attitude, increased spiritual and body awareness
- Happiness!

Let's jump right in and talk about some important aspects of the kidney cleanse. Here are some specifics about the juice feast and the kidney cleanse teas and herbs. (See the next chapter for details about the kidney cleanse food plan.)

THE 3-DAY JUICE FEAST

"Juice feasting" is essentially juice fasting, but I believe that the positive phrase is much more empowering than the negative. Therefore, I'm using the term "juice feast" rather than "juice fast," because the amount of fresh produce you will be consuming daily in no way resembles a true fast, which requires abstinence from all food and liquids. Although you won't be chewing on any meats, breads, or roughage, you will be taking in more high-quality nutrients than you've ever consumed in a single day.

You will have an abundance of freshly made vegetable and fruit juice blends, herbal teas, and broths filled with highly available vitamins, minerals, antioxidants, phytochemicals, and enzymes. Your body can utilize these nutrients therapeutically to remove toxins while also supporting the repair of tissues.

One of the beautiful things about a juice feast is that, without the need for major digestion, your body can spend its resources on healing and cleansing. Basically, you are allowing your body to go on the offense, clearing stubborn and stagnant waste that otherwise wouldn't be removed. Think of it this way: Imagine you are in bed with the flu, barely able to move, and your house is a mess. You know you need to do the dishes, wash the pile of clothes lying on the floor, and clear away the mess, but you don't, you just can't. You don't have the motivation or the energy to do it, so your house remains dirty.

This is your body on a day-to-day basis: so inundated with toxins that it cannot do anything other than use every resource it has just to stay afloat. It has neither the physical energy nor the nutrients to expend moving old stagnant toxins or to repair damaged tissue.

Now, imagine that the next day the flu has lifted and you feel better. You got 12 hours of rest, drank plenty of water, and knocked that nasty bug out. You look around the house and suddenly your perspective changes. You are ready and willing to clean up your mess and get your house organized, so you do it and soon the house is immaculate!

This is your body on the juice feast. A detoxifying environment is now perfectly in place: Your body has the nutrients to provide energy to cells to push toxins out, and it has access to therapeutic cleansing agents to pull the toxins out. With the support of the liver, these toxins are neutralized and passed either to the kidneys or the bowels for elimination.

WHY 3 DAYS?

It is generally accepted that 3 days of juice feasting is the ideal duration needed for the body to optimally detoxify. The body is a complicated organism and does not follow our philosophy of instant gratification. Change takes time. In 3 days the body has a real chance to start making a change, which will be solidified in the following weeks of the cleanse. However, depending on your state of health, your history with fasting, and your mental relationship with food, you may be able to complete only 1 full day of juice feasting—but, remember, the juice feast is not the full cleanse. It is followed by a 3-week food plan that further cleanses and repairs the body. So, even if you do just 1 day of feasting, you will still reap enormous benefits from the kidney cleanse.

ARE ALL JUICES THE SAME?

It is imperative that the juice you consume during the juice feast is freshly made. This means either making the juice at home or purchasing it from a juice store or health food store. When buying, make sure the juice is freshly made, and if pre-bottled that it was made with a hydraulic press juicer. When juice is bottled, its nutrients begin to degrade, lessening its ability to cleanse the body. The exception is juice made with a hydraulic press juicer, because this juicing method maintains nutrient content for up to 3 days.

Regular store-bought juices are not acceptable for the juice feast. Most are made from concentrates rather than fresh-pressed fruits and vegetables. What this means is they do not contain the life-providing nutrients and energies necessary to cleanse the body. In addition, store-bought juices are almost always pasteurized. Pasteurization is the process that kills any enzymes present in the juice while degrading the nutrients—which is counterproductive, since the nutrients and enzymes in juice are needed for cleansing the body. Furthermore, store-bought juice is full of excess sugar that actually inhibits the cleansing process and promotes the growth of harmful pathogens such as fungi and bacteria. The bottom line is that you should make your own juice or purchase it from a local source that makes fresh-pressed juice.

GREEN JUICES VS. FRUIT JUICES

This kidney cleanse focuses on fresh vegetable juices, specifically green juices, with a minimal amount of fruit juices. Green juices are the best of all juices because green leafy vegetables and herbs are highest in nutrients and detoxifying agents. Also, green vegetables contain chlorophyll, which provides a laundry list of benefits to the body ranging from blood building to improving liver detoxification.

The reason to focus on vegetable juices is not just because green juices are so nutrient dense, which promotes more rapid detoxification, but also because fruit juices contain fructose. Fructose is a naturally occurring sugar that in high levels can cause blood sugar imbalances as well as act as fuel for bad guys such as fungi and bacteria. Therefore, the juice feast uses low-sugar fruits sparingly, with the exception of a few fruits (watermelon, pineapple, oranges) that have particularly high healing and cleansing properties for the kidneys.

Note: If you currently suffer from or have passed calcium oxalate stones, please refer to the chapter "Special Programs" (page 123). Many green vegetables contain high levels of oxalates, which increase the formation of kidney stones in people who have previously formed calcium oxalate stones.

POTATO JUICE: During the kidney cleanse you will be incorporating potato juice from organic russet potatoes. Potatoes contain high levels of potassium citrate, an alkaline salt used as a non-irritating diuretic that helps cleanse the kidneys. It is widely used to treat kidney stones by preventing the formation of mineral crystals in the kidney. Potassium citrate also prevents the urine from becoming acidic, which helps to prevent uric acid and cystine from accumulating in the kidneys. While potassium citrate is necessary for those who have a history of kidney stones, its effects on the kidney are beneficial for anyone looking to improve kidney health.

ORGANIC VS. CONVENTIONAL PRODUCE

Here is the bottom line: If I had my way, you would use 100% organic produce to avoid exposure to any pesticides, herbicides, GMOs (genetically modified foods), or fungicides during this cleanse. After all, the goal is to reduce your overall toxic load so that your body can focus on detoxifying and healing. But I realize that we do not live in a perfect world and not everyone will have access or the means to purchase 100% organic produce. So, let's implement the "second best" rule when needed.

Purchase organic when possible, but using conventional is not a deal breaker. Fortunately, fruits and vegetables contain an array of antioxidants that help to clear many of the toxins that may be present in conventional produce, so the benefits outweigh the disadvantages. If you are using conventional produce, be sure to wash it thoroughly and to peel the skins off fruits.

You can also use the "Organic/Conventional Shopping Guide" on page 219 to prioritize which produce should be organic because it is highly sprayed with pesticides (dirty), and which produce is not sprayed (clean) and is okay grown conventionally.

KIDNEY CLEANSE TEAS

Every day you will be drinking teas made from the herbs corn silk and dandelion. These therapeutic herbs promote kidney health and ease physiological change.

I know what you may be thinking: Why do I need to drink herb teas when I am doing the juice feast and am on the kidney cleanse food plan? It seems like too much trouble to worry about drinking tea all day, especially when tea is for the British and for old Chinese men with long white beards, right? The truth is that if you want this cleanse to work, and I mean really work, then you will have to drink the tea. Whether that involves a one-way ticket to China or joining a British tea appreciation club, you gotta do it.

Herbs have been an integral part of medicine for thousands of years. Using plants and plant substances to treat all kinds of diseases and medical conditions is thought to have originated in prehistoric times. Ancient Chinese and Egyptian writings describe medicinal uses for plants as early as 3000 BC, and researchers have found that people in different parts of the world tend to use the same or similar plants for the same purposes. Herbs are the foundation of remedies from Chinese and Ayurvedic medicine, and historically they have been used to create pharmaceutical drugs in Western medicine. The University of Maryland asserts that almost one-fourth of current pharmaceutical drugs are derived from botanicals. A few examples are digoxin (foxglove), morphine (poppy), ephedrine (*Ephedra sinica*), and Taxol (*Taxus brevifolia*, or Pacific yew).

While the kidney cleanse food plan is a very powerful and indispensable tool, it is the herbs that most efficiently change the biochemistry of the body. That is why herbs are also referred to as botanical medicines or phytomedicines. The nice thing about herbs compared with drugs is that they have the ability to work on the root of a problem rather than just address the symptoms. They provide the body with the substances that promote long-lasting changes. Alternative and holistic practitioners love using herbs instead of pharmaceutical drugs because they are often much gentler on the body and don't elicit the same potentially toxic side effects.

Note: Because herbs are not regulated with the same scrutiny as pharmaceutical drugs, it is vital for you to do your own research to be sure you get safe, clean products. Herbs can have interactions with pharmaceutical drugs or have adverse effects on various health conditions, so consult your doctor first.

KIDNEY CLEANSE HERBS

Although many herbs are known to promote kidney health, this cleanse focuses on corn silk and dandelion, which have a wealth of scientific and clinical evidence supporting their effectiveness. For example, in Germany, dandelion is licensed as a standard medicinal tea to stimulate urination. In addition, both corn silk and dandelion are generally recognized as safe—which is very important, since many herbs used in other kidney cleansing programs have side effects and can potentially harm the kidneys.

Corn Silk (*Zea mays*)

A traditional herbal medicine, corn silk is recognized worldwide as a soothing diuretic. It also has been used as a remedy for urinary conditions including urinary tract infections, edema, kidney stones, and bladder infections, and as a lymphatic cleanser. It soothes and relaxes the lining of the bladder and urinary tubules, thus reducing irritation and promoting urination. In addition, corn silk is an excellent antioxidant, protecting against the poisonous effects of toxins on the kidneys.

An interesting study indicates that corn silk modifies glomerular function (remember, the glomuleri filter waste from the blood) and potassium urinary excretion, thereby reducing the risk of kidney stones and increasing the kidneys' ability to filter waste. Another study demonstrates that corn silk increases the contraction of the smooth muscles of the ureter, leading to an increase in urinary output and the passing of waste products. Finally, a study done on rabbits suffering from nephrocalcinosis (calcium deposits that reduce kidney function) showed that corn silk helped restore some kidney function by accelerating calcium and waste excretion.

The active components of corn silk are as follows: essential oils (carvacrol, alpha-terpineol, menthol, and thymol), flavonoids (maysin), saponins, tannins, sterols, and alkaloids. Corn silk also contains 1,8-cineole, beta-carotene, beta-sitosterol, geraniol, hordenine, limonene, niacin, riboflavin, selenium, vitamin C, and vitexin.

Dandelion (*Taraxacum officinale*)

Dandelion leaves have been used extensively as a kidney treatment in traditional folk medicine and modern-day phytotherapy (the use of plants or plant extracts for medical purposes). It has proved its efficacy in many research studies. Possibly because of its potassium content, dandelion has an alkalizing effect on urine and is often used to reduce urinary tract "gravel" and to prevent kidney stones, which can develop from the gravel. Dandelion's effectiveness is believed to stem from its saponin and flavone content, which also contributes to its antimicrobial effects.

The active components of dandelion are as follows: bitter taraxacins (eudesmanolides), sitosterol, stigmasterol, alpha- and beta-carotene, caffeic acid, mucilage, flavone, saponin, and an unusually high potassium content. Dandelion also contains vitamins A, C, D, and B complex as well as iron, magnesium, zinc, manganese, copper, choline, calcium, boron, and silicon.

I'll tell you up front that at least 75% of the work needed to successfully complete this cleanse must be done before you actually begin the cleanse program. Preparation is everything when you embark on something new, especially when it has to do with your health. During the cleanse, you'll be making changes in the way you conduct your day-to-day routine, how you interact socially, how you view yourself, and how you prioritize your health. I realize these changes are not always easy, especially if you are a creature of habit like me, and that is why it's important to prepare by getting your house in order.

PLANNING AND PREPARING MENTALLY

Unlike most cleanses, which ask you simply to take a few supplements out of a box or drink some juice for a few days, this cleanse requires a bit more from you. I am not saying this cleanse is complicated, because it isn't, but I am saying that you must be mentally prepared and present. You will see that this is a good thing, as this is where real change happens—and I believe that you are reading this book because you are ready for change.

So, what do you do to plan and prepare mentally? I am convinced that the best way is to know why you are doing this cleanse. If you don't know why you are doing something, how are you ever going to have enough motivation to follow through, especially when you come up against temptations? Think cheesy pizza, late-night ice cream sessions, or buttery popcorn and candy at the movies.

I want you to create a word processing document, grab a journal, or even pull a sheet of lined paper from your kid's binder and title it, "My Health Goals." Then really think about what you want to accomplish with this cleanse and how you would like to feel both physically and mentally. Here are a few goals I've jotted down in the past:

- Feel energized all day long without the need for caffeine
- Have a clear head capable of being focused and driven
- Get rid of low back pain—feel limber and flexible
- Eliminate feelings of fear and anxiety, be ready to tackle any obstacle
- Have thick and shiny hair, strong and fast-growing nails
- Build a strong immune system free of disease and illness

Now date and sign it after adding the following pledge:

"I am ready and willing to do whatever it takes to ensure that I achieve my health goals. I deserve to feel radiantly healthy, free of all disease, symptoms, and illness."

I want you to look at your list of goals and your pledge at least once a week (every morning is ideal). This will remind you why you are doing this cleanse, why you are dedicating your valuable time, energy, and money to your health, and how you are at that very moment actively transforming your health. With this daily reminder, you are sending your subconscious a message that will eventually become part of your being and your way of living. This is key to staying motivated throughout the cleanse and harnessing the power to make permanent life changes, especially when staying on track may seem difficult.

THE EMOTIONAL JOURNEY

One of the greatest things you will take away from this cleanse is a new insight into your body and your emotions, because food is often intimately tied to feelings. We eat to fill the void of sadness or loneliness, we eat to reward ourselves or to celebrate, we eat to remind ourselves of better times. Each one of these emotions is fueled by a perceived emotional satisfaction and not by hunger. When you start eliminating foods used as an emotional crutch, your body may react, perhaps in full-blown rebellion. By forcing yourself to no longer rely on these foods during the cleanse, you'll achieve a new level of growth, allowing you to recognize the emotions and feelings that arise in their absence.

With that recognition, you can begin to seek, identify, and understand why you are feeling the way you do. Once you do this, you have the choice to begin finding alternative methods for filling those same emotional needs—and that's a very powerful tool in your health journey.

I am not saying that you cannot use food as a means of creating an emotional experience, but rather that you shouldn't rely on it. It is that dependency that keeps a person from being able to make healthy food choices in the long run. Once you get to the root of the dependency, you can gain control over it, and you can make decisions on whether or not to indulge mindfully, in a manner that is no longer harmful to body or mind.

DEALING WITH JUICE FEASTING

I want to take a moment to talk specifically about the juice feast, because the emotional process I just laid out will most likely come up during these 3 days. I am not going to tell you that it's a breeze to subsist on juice for 3 days as all the raw foodies and celebrities claim—because it is not, especially if you are new to this practice. It is a challenge, about 85% emotional and 15% physical. I will tell you how the story ends. You will live on juice for 3 days, you will not starve, and, no, you will not die. You will be in awe of yourself, as if you had just climbed Everest. You will feel completely empowered.

In an attempt to gently guide you through this emotional surge, I have placed the juice feast at the beginning of the cleanse. I have found that the greatest chance of success comes when facing the biggest challenge up front, when the motivation and dedication to begin something new are strongest. You will notice that the strictest guidelines come at the beginning of the cleanse, because that forces you to overcome flooding emotions that might cause you to quit or "cheat." By completing a 3-day juice feast up front, you will be well on your way to a successful cleanse.

SETTING ASIDE TIME FOR THE CLEANSE AND YOUR HEALTH

Now that you have decided to embark on this cleansing journey, the next step is to plan the time do it. I do not want you to read this book and then jump right into the cleanse the next day, because you need to plan. The planning process will depend on where you are in your health journey. Some of you will already be implementing some aspects of the cleanse, while for others cleansing may be a brand-new concept. Based on where you are on your journey, set aside between a couple of hours to a full day for preparation.

To give you an overview of the changes I am talking about, the following is a list of preparation tasks. If there is something on the list that you are already doing, you can skip over it. As for the rest of you, here are the tasks in a nutshell so there are absolutely no surprises, and therefore no excuses. Remember that success lies in your ability to mentally prepare and be organized for what is to come. Please do not take the preparation period lightly.

GROCERY SHOPPING: Once or twice a week you will have to sit down and make a list of food items needed for the cleanse. I recommend creating a meal schedule of the recipes you will be making that week. From that, you can write a list of the ingredients needed.

In all likelihood, not all of the ingredients that you need to prepare foods and juices for the cleanse will be available at the market you are used to going to, so check out local health food stores and farmer's markets. Shopping at a local farmer's market will be very helpful to you during the cleanse. Browsing through rows of freshly picked produce and speaking with the farmers can be extremely inspiring and makes the process of eating healthy foods that much more fun and delicious. So if you don't typically shop at a farmer's market or have never been to one before, this is an excellent time to start.

Time needed: You need time to decide which recipes to make, to compile a shopping list, and to shop. Do not underestimate the importance of this part of your preparation. If you try to wing it by going to the market at the last minute without a list or recipes to follow, hoping to buy the right foods, you are setting yourself up for failure. Invest in success.

JUICING AND SMOOTHIE MAKING: If you are new to juicing and smoothie making, this process can be a bit intimidating. The concept of washing and chopping vegetables and fruits, blending or juicing, and then cleaning the blender or juicer can seem overwhelming. Acknowledge that it is going to take a little time, and factor that into your day. Do a test run on the weekend to see how long it takes, and based on that, either get up a bit earlier in the morning or take some time on the weekend to prep. You can always wash and chop fruits and vegetables ahead of time to make the process go faster.

Time needed: See how long it takes you to prep the ingredients, blend or juice, and clean up. I can do all of it in less than 15 minutes, and that's with prepping everything each morning. Find out what works for you and be prepared to incorporate that amount of time into your day.

PREPARING AND COOKING FOOD: I know many of you cringe at the thought of getting in the kitchen and cooking your own food. But guess what? It is time to overcome that fear and to tackle it head on, because at this point in your life, you're the only one you can trust to prepare the foods you need to live a long and healthy life.

Most of the recipes in the book do not take much longer than 30 minutes to make, and I know you can fit that time into your day if you are dedicated. The recipes are easy to put together, and you will not have to figure out how to do complicated things like make a soufflé. However, I know that "life happens" and that some things are out of your control, so I have given you a lifeline—a good guide for dining out. This will involve utilizing the food lists in the reference section to customize meals so that no matter the location you can stay on course with the cleanse.

Time needed: Decide on the recipes you want to make the next day, read the instructions, and determine how much time you will need for preparation. If you work away from home, don't forget to include the time to prepare a lunch to take with you.

MAKING TIME FOR ADJUNCT THERAPIES: With this cleanse, you will be using adjunct therapies, such as dry brushing, castor oil packs, and saunas, to support the cleansing process. You will have to make the time to fit these into your busy schedule, but keep in mind that they are not practices used only while cleansing the kidneys. They are cleansing practices that you can continue as part of your lifelong health and wellness routine. Taking the time to learn how to do them now will be very helpful in the long run.

Time needed: Set aside time to get the necessary tools to perform the therapy at home or find a local place to have the therapy performed for you. And, of course, you have to make the time to actually do them. These therapies can take from 5 minutes to 1 hour. The good thing is that they are like a special treat during the cleansing process—super relaxing and invigorating!

TALKING TO YOUR FRIENDS AND FAMILY

Your friends and family can either be your best allies or your worst enemies. In my experience, it's typically the latter. While many of us dream that we can do this cleanse with our partners, best friends, and family members, most often it's just that—a dream. It's essential that you take the time to sort out your stance and feelings about undergoing this cleanse, because I will tell you now that one of the hardest parts about taking charge of your health and wellness could be pushback from loved ones.

The best advice I can give you is that if you feel secure in your decision, then even the worst naysayers cannot break your will. I recommend that you sit down and think about how you want to talk about this cleanse, because solidifying your phrasing is key. You want to be able to speak clearly and directly about why you are cleansing and why it is important to you so that your message is heard and respected.

There are typically two ways of addressing this issue. You can decide to talk openly to your friends and family, asking them to respect your decision, or you can decide to not talk about it, thereby avoiding any negative feedback or peer pressure. But if you do choose to talk about it, then you are responsible to others for completing the cleanse. Either way, make a decision before you begin the cleanse so that you are not caught off guard and your determination isn't compromised.

On a positive note, if you do find a friend or family member to do the cleanse with you, all the better! Having someone to juice with, dine with, and share experiences with is invaluable to your success, especially in the long run. If you have someone in mind, don't be afraid to ask that person to join you!

DEALING WITH SOCIAL ENGAGEMENTS

From personal experience I know that social engagements can make cleansing difficult. Although cleansing is becoming more widely accepted, making it more of a valid excuse for not wanting to share that cheesy appetizer or indulging in a large margarita at happy hour, that does not always get you off the hook. There will be birthday parties, holidays, family dinners, sporting events, and office meetings typically centered around naughty indulgent behaviors that are on the "avoid" list for the kidney cleanse. So, how exactly are you going to maintain your social calendar while on the cleanse?

Plan accordingly. If Thanksgiving and Christmas are coming up and you know that there is no way you are going to opt out of pumpkin pie, sugar cookies, and eggnog, then starting the kidney cleanse at this time is not the best idea. Wait a month or so until you know you will be able to dedicate yourself to cleansing.

As for typical social engagements, you have a couple of options. Always do your research. If you are planning on going to a restaurant, check the menu ahead of time and decide if the menu options fit with the kidney cleanse food plan. If it does, plan what you are going to order in advance, and stick to it. On the other hand, if the menu offers no acceptable options, either eat beforehand or gently suggest another restaurant. You don't have to explain your predicament—simply recommend another restaurant that you heard had great reviews. No need to come off as being difficult.

If you are dining at someone's home, I suggest calling ahead to see what's on the menu. A great way to do this without prying is to offer to bring something. That way you "need" to know what is on the menu. Then you can decide if there is something being served that you can eat. If there are no options that fit the cleanse, eat something beforehand. At the dinner, you can find the least offensive foods and eat small portions of them.

Finally, there will be some events where the best option is to politely decline—I am thinking of something like a football party with beer pong and other celebratory drinking games. At such events there will be nothing suitable for you to eat and peer pressure may be just too strong for you to resist.

Remember, with a little preparation there is almost always a way to maintain your social calendar while still cleansing. Your experience at a party or dinner may be a little different than usual, but you still will have the best of both worlds.

CHAPTER FIVE

THE KIDNEY CLEANSE FOOD PLAN

Don't be scared off by the thought of a food plan. This is not a diet, where the focus is on what's taken away—this food plan focuses on what is gained. As you've have learned in previous chapters, the kidneys are very powerful, yet vulnerable to physical stress and must be protected. The number-one cause of stress is from what we eat, so we must be conscious of what we put in our mouths.

Everything that goes into the body must be broken down, assimilated, neutralized, filtered, and possibly eliminated. I know, you don't want to think about that part and would rather concentrate on the part where the food tastes good—but when it comes to working on your health, thinking beyond the basics is important.

For example, steak may not seem like a big deal to consume, but to the body it is a huge deal. The digestive track has to do a lot of work to break down the steak (metabolize it), in the process using up vital energy that could be used for other functions. If the steak doesn't break down properly, the result is toxic byproducts, including some of the big bullies such as urea, ammonia, and uric acid, which essentially beat up the kidneys. The presence of toxic byproducts causes the kidneys to work harder, which means that the other jobs the kidneys must perform take a back seat. In turn, clinical symptoms such as scanty urine, low back pain, and sometimes a gradual increase in blood pressure occur. It's all connected.

The aim of the kidney cleanse food plan is to greatly reduce or eliminate stress on the kidneys caused by toxic end products from food. The kidneys can then focus on clearing old waste products, and the tissues can begin to rebuild using healing foods. Everything on the food plan is rich in nutrients that promote detoxification and support the intricate processes of kidney function. Each of the foods was chosen with these parameters in mind, so you will be in good hands!

In addition to consuming outrageously healthy kidney foods, you will also be focusing on how to eat them.

First, you will be drinking only "superfood" smoothies for breakfast. Superfoods are nutrient powerhouses packed with vitamins, minerals, antioxidants, and other healthful substances. Starting the day with a liquid meal allows the body to focus on detoxifying rather than digesting, and it also provides a boost of nutrients to support the natural cleansing and rebuilding functions of the kidneys for the day.

Second, it will be your goal to eat dinner at least 3 hours before bedtime. This is important because if you consume food any later, the food won't have time to digest properly, leaving it to rot. The result is that more toxins are created, which leads to stress on the kidneys.

THE FOOD PLAN AND KIDNEY FUNCTION

To make the concept of eating for kidney health clearer, let's start by reviewing the main functions of the kidneys. Here's what the kidneys do: regulate pH balance and water and electrolyte balance; maintain blood pressure by managing water volume, sodium, and hormone production; filter and excrete toxins and metabolic waste products; convert a precursor vitamin to vitamin D; and stimulate red blood cell production.

I don't expect you to memorize this, but referring to this is going to be really useful in understanding why a substance affects the kidneys positively or negatively. If it negatively impacts a kidney function, then we are going to eliminate the substance. If it improves kidney function, then we are going to keep it. Simple as that.

Let's look at how the acidity or alkalinity (pH) of various foods affects the kidneys. Then let's consider how water figures in and whether or not salt is good or bad for health.

ACID OR ALKALINE?

The kidneys work constantly to maintain the perfect pH balance, and the more you do to minimize fluctuations, the more you allow the kidneys to focus on clearing toxins. But how can you help pH balance? The answer is simple: by consuming predominantly alkalizing foods.

According to Robert Young, Ph.D., author of *The pH Miracle*, all ingested foods release electrons as well as leave an ash residue when they break down. This ash residue can be neutral, acidic, or alkaline, depending on the mineral content of the food. Alkaline foods provide the body with electrons (used for energy), whereas acidic foods remove electrons. And if electron content determines a food's alkalinity, then you want to consume foods that contain lots of electrons.

In general, animal protein (meat, eggs, and dairy), processed and refined foods, fermented foods, grains, artificial sweeteners, sweet fruits, and sugars are acidifying, as are alcohol, coffee, black tea, chocolate, and soda. On the other hand, vegetables, sour citrus fruits, essential fatty acids, and sprouted nuts, seeds, and grains are alkalizing. Fruits and vegetables contain organic, naturally occurring sodium, which binds with bicarbonate. This sodium bicarbonate buffers (neutralizes) acid, thereby alkalinizing the body. Foods such as animal protein cause more acid to be formed in the cells, and over time the excess acid overwhelms the body's buffering system, leaving the body depleted of valuable minerals (sodium, potassium, and calcium) and causing higher levels of acid to be excreted by the kidneys.

This does not mean all acidifying foods are a no-no. It just means you will consume mostly alkalizing ones and a few of the less acidifying foods in moderation.

THE BONE LOSS-PH CONNECTION

One of the main underlying causes of bone loss (osteoporosis and osteopenia) is acidic pH. When the body becomes acidic due to high levels of toxins, stress, and the consumption of acidic foods such as animal protein, sugars, and fried foods, the body must search for minerals to alkalinize the pH. First the body looks to soft tissue reserves. If minerals are present, the body uses them—but when none are present, which is common in people with chronic acidic pH, the body takes minerals from the bones. This process sets the stage for bone loss, because the minerals pulled from the bone cause the breakdown of the bones themselves.

Once the blood is alkalinized with minerals from the bones, we often have leftover calcium that cannot be deposited back into the bones. What does the body do with that calcium? It deposits it in other areas of the body such as the kidneys, the eyes, and the cardiovascular system. Furthermore, because the body often balances acidic urinary pH by leaching calcium from the bones, this further promotes the formation of kidney stones. The goal of promoting alkalinity in the body will not only improve kidney health and reduce the risk of stone formation, but will also improve bone density. Look at that! Two birds, one stone.

WHAT ARE THE TOP ALKALIZING FOODS?

To get the most bang for the buck, you are going to focus on consuming plenty of the top alkalizing foods (those that contain the most electrons) to balance out some of the more acidic foods you will be eating. The following is Dr. Young's top list.

1. CHLOROPHYLL: Green vegetables and grasses (oat, wheat, barley)

2. ESSENTIAL FATTY ACIDS: Flax, chia seeds, hemp, olives, raw nuts and seeds, avocados, borage, and evening primrose

3. PURIFIED WATER

4. UNREFINED SEA SALT

Note: You may notice that many kidney superfoods (page 62) are in the acidic category, but if you eat them in balance with enough alkaline foods, you will still be able to promote an alkaline pH.

WATER — THE ESSENCE OF LIFE, THE KEY TO KIDNEY HEALTH

Without water, there is no life. Plants cannot live without it, animals cannot live without it, and certainly we are no exception to the rule. The human body consists of up to 60% water. Blood is 83 to 92% water, the brain and muscles are 75% water, and bones are about 22% water. It is clear that water is essential to our very makeup.

Clean water is critical to wellness, and staying hydrated is the single most effective way to cleanse your kidneys and maintain optimal health. Remember, the kidneys are in charge of flushing toxins out of the body via urine, and urine is 95% water. So, how can your kidneys flush out toxins without proper hydration? You're right, they can't. Staying hydrated is mandatory for this cleanse. No ifs, ands, or buts, and certainly no substitutions.

Here's the bottom line: Without adequate clean water, your kidneys can't function properly. There is no way around this fact. Even if the only thing you took away from this book is to drink more water, I would be happy. The truth is that by simply increasing your water intake you will start seeing improvements in health. No water, no happy kidneys. You should be drinking enough water so that your urine is light yellow and you are urinating between 6 and 10 times a day.

How do you know how much water is enough? The general rule is to drink half your weight in ounces of water a day. This does not include water contained in any other beverage. I am talking about pure water only. Keep in mind that the half-your-weight recommendation is a baseline. Factors that will increase your need for extra water include exercising, living in a hot climate, and drinking dehydrating beverages such as tea and coffee. The rule is that for every cup of coffee or caffeinated tea you consume, you have to add 16 ounces of water to your total water requirement for the day. Since coffee or tea are out for the duration of the kidney cleanse, you won't have to compensate for that.

I recommend that you drink room-temperature water, not cold water or ice water. This is a foundational rule from Chinese and Ayurvedic medicine and is based on the idea that cold water and other liquids cause the constriction of blood vessels and nerves in the stomach. Digestion calls for heat and metabolic energy (yang), and cold inhibits the process. Cold water leads to improper digestion and weakened kidneys since the body must use the yang/fire energy from the kidneys to aid in heating the stomach.

Facts about dehydration:

- Mild dehydration can slow metabolism.
- Dehydration is the number-one cause of daytime fatigue.

- A 3% drop in water causes a 10% drop in muscle strength and an 8% drop in speed.
- Improper hydration causes short-term memory problems, anxiety, irritability, and depression.
- Dehydration may cause sugar cravings.
- Mild dehydration is associated with acid reflux, migraines, constipation, fibromyalgia, and colitis. Severe dehydration is associated with diabetes, heart disease, allergies, high blood pressure, asthma, and cancer.

Recommendation: Drink half your weight in ounces of purified water a day.

FILTERED WATER

I recommend that you purchase a water filtration system for your home. Whether it's a full-house system (ideal) or just a pitcher with a filter, you will get a much cleaner, safe alternative to both bottled water and tap water. The ideal system is a reverse-osmosis or ionizing filtration system. Since you will be drinking plenty of water during this cleanse, I urge you to follow this advice.

I also recommend against drinking hard water because it contains lots of minerals, especially calcium, which plays a role in kidney stone formation. If you have hard water at home, look for a water softener to install.

SALT: TO EAT OR NOT TO EAT?

Salt is at the top of every doctor's list of items to stay away from when dealing with kidney problems, especially high blood pressure—and that advice is not without reason. Sodium chloride, or table salt, is a highly refined and manufactured product that may induce stress on the mineral balance of the body, leading to a host of health problems. But is all salt to blame or is it merely common table salt? And if salt generally is so terrible, how do you explain sea salt taking over the shelves of health food stores across the nation?

WHY IS SALT IMPORTANT TO THE KIDNEYS?

As you now know, the kidneys control fluid and electrolyte balance, filter waste products, and regulate blood pressure. Sodium, the main component of salt, is a vital player in all these functions. So, salt—the right kind of salt and the proper amount of it—is an extremely important player in maintaining kidney health. Let's look at salt's three key roles in kidney function.

1. SOURCE OF ENERGY FOR REABSORPTION AND SECRETION: A key function of the kidneys is to filter waste products and to hold onto important nutrients from the blood through the process of reabsorption and secretion. Sodium makes this process possible.

2. BLOOD VOLUME AND PRESSURE: The kidneys control blood volume and pressure by adjusting the level of sodium. When blood volume or pressure decreases, the kidneys reabsorb sodium (and release potassium), resulting in an increase in blood volume and return of pressure to normal levels.

3. MAINTAINING FLUID BALANCE: Since the body is predominantly water, the regulation of fluids is important to health, making the kidneys' role vital. Sodium plays a significant part because water goes where sodium goes. When the body needs to increase water volume, it holds onto sodium, and when it needs to reduce water volume, it releases sodium.

UNREFINED SEA SALT VS. REFINED TABLE SALT

The difference between unrefined sea salt (the good guy) and refined table salt (the bad guy) all comes down to two things: chemistry and additives.

The chemistry of the two types of salt differs. Table salt is void of trace minerals such as potassium, magnesium, and calcium, which are imperative for the chemical actions of sodium chloride in the body. Without the trace minerals, sodium chloride causes imbalances in the body systems and may lead to negative health effects. In contrast, sea salt contains these valuable trace minerals essential to the proper functioning of body systems.

Because table salt has been refined, it doesn't easily combine with human body fluid, which undermines the most basic chemical and metabolic processes in the body. Table salt prevents the free crossing of liquids and minerals, causing fluids to accumulate and stagnate in the joints, lymphatic ducts, lymph nodes, and kidneys. In addition, table salt contains additives that may be undesirable to the body, forcing the body's systems to eliminate them and leading to additional stress on the eliminatory systems. It is then no wonder that table salt can lead to health problems, making it a valid item to eliminate from the diet, especially while on the kidney cleanse.

WHAT ABOUT THE NEGATIVE EFFECTS OF SALT?

We know through countless studies that too much sodium leads to stress on the kidneys as well as the body generally because it puts the delicate balancing mechanisms into hyper drive. When the body is under stress, things can go awry: high blood pressure, osteoporosis, kidney stones, acid pH, heart disease, and even possibly gastric cancer. But it should be noted that these studies were conducted with refined salt, which lacks the trace minerals to balance sodium chloride. The question remains: Is it the high intake of refined sodium that leads to kidney stress and disease, or is it the high intake of salt in general?

While I haven't found any research studies on this topic, I submit that it is refined table salt that leads to kidney stress and disease, not unrefined sea salt. I am not saying consume loads of sea salt without moderation, but I am saying that the incorporation of unrefined sea salt is imperative for health and will not be stressful with a plant-based diet rich in potassium.

THE SALT CONCLUSION

Unrefined sea salt in, refined table salt out.

Not only does unrefined sea salt provide the energy to properly move waste products out of the blood for excretion, but it maintains proper fluid balance to flush the toxins out. It also helps the body to maintain proper pH, and it is the raw material used by the kidneys for many of its daily functions. Given these benefits, it's imperative to use unrefined sea salt and to eliminate refined table salt. Unrefined sea salt is used in the delicious recipes in this book, including the recipes for juices and smoothies.

General recommendation: ¼–1 teaspoon of unrefined sea salt daily

Note: For those of you dealing with a kidney disease or condition, I am not recommending that you incorporate unrefined sea salt into your diet. Consult your doctor about salt use.

KIDNEY-SPECIFIC FOODS

We all know that certain foods are healthy based on their ability to provide valuable nutrients such as vitamins, minerals, antioxidants, and amino acids. Let's look even further and focus on the foods that are essential for the kidneys to function optimally as well as enhance their detoxification capability. Since the main mechanism for cleansing the kidneys is increased dilution and thus urination, a number of the foods in the kidney cleanse food plan are diuretics, which promote urination. The more you can increase the water load in the kidneys, the more you can dilute harmful toxins and flush them out.

Other foods that are beneficial for cleansing the kidneys are those with anti-inflammatory properties, antimicrobial properties, and a high antioxidant content. Because the kidneys are very susceptible to damage from toxins, whether from chemicals, microbes, or even the end products of digestion, it's very important to offset that damage with these agents. When congestion occurs in the kidneys, inflammation is a response, further inhibiting kidney function. Therefore, we are going to use every trick possible to help the kidneys.

To review, many of the foods in the kidney cleanse food plan have one or more of the following qualities:

- Antilithic (acts against formation of kidney and other stones)
- Antiseptic (prevents growth of disease-causing organisms)
- Antihepatotoxic (cleanses the blood)
- Antinephrotoxic (neutralizes kidney toxins)
- Diuretic (increases passage of urine)
- Anti-inflammatory (reduces inflammation)

- Antioxidant (removes damaging oxidizing agents)
- Restorative

Note: The superfoods listed below are recommended for people with healthy kidneys. If you are dealing with any disease of the kidneys, see the "Special Programs" chapter on page 123.

KIDNEY SUPERFOODS

APPLE CIDER VINEGAR, RAW (UNPASTEURIZED): Rich in minerals and acetic acid, apple cider vinegar promotes kidney cleansing by stimulating proper digestion. In studies, it has been shown to lower systolic blood pressure (the first, higher number) and balance blood glucose.

ASPARAGUS: Known for its diuretic effects on the body, asparagus promotes filtration by the kidneys. It promotes the clearance of oxalic crystals from the kidneys, thereby reducing the incidence of kidney stones.

BEETS: High levels of nutrients in beets, such as iron, vitamin C, B vitamins, calcium, magnesium, and phosphorus, support the kidneys and the blood. These nutrients are also imperative for liver and gallbladder detoxification, which reduces the body's overall toxic load. Beets are rich in organic sodium, which promotes mineral and fluid balance in the kidneys.

BLACK/TART CHERRIES: Black and tart cherries are beneficial for promoting the clearance of uric acid and reducing inflammation in the kidneys. Uric acid plays a role in kidney stone development and the inflammatory condition called gout.

CAYENNE: The active ingredient in cayenne, capsaicin, has been shown to protect against toxin-induced kidney damage in people treated with the chemotherapy drug cisplatin. It also has shown to protect against damage to lipids, the delicate fats in the kidneys.

CELERY: The fact that celery is high in chlorophyll makes it an excellent blood cleanser. Celery is also high in organic sodium, which supports kidney function and the movement of lymphatic fluid. The chlorophyll and nutrient content promote an alkaline pH. Celery has traditionally been used as a natural diuretic and for lowering blood pressure. In one study, celery demonstrated its ability to boost the excretion of urinary calcium, thereby reducing the incidence of kidney stones.

CRANBERRIES: This fruit has long been valued for its antimicrobial properties and its ability to protect against urinary tract infections. One of the most common ways to get a kidney infection is through transmission from the urinary tract. Therefore, maintaining a healthy urinary tract is important to kidney health.

Studies have shown that cranberries prevent urinary tract infections in two different ways. The first is by making the urine more acidic, and bacteria grow best in an alkaline environment. The second way was revealed in a study done by the Weizman Institute of Science and Tel Aviv University, which found evidence that cranberries prevented bacteria from attaching to the bladder wall.

Note: Cranberries are not recommended for anyone prone to calcium oxalate stones, because they contain oxalates.

CUCUMBERS: In addition to being a natural diuretic, cucumbers promote an alkaline pH and excretion of waste products such as uric acid. They are a natural source of potassium and magnesium, which makes them a key food for maintaining blood pressure. Because they consist mainly of water, cucumbers are extremely hydrating.

FLAXSEEDS: Flaxseeds are more than just a good source of plant-based protein. Studies indicate that they reduce the excretion of protein via the urine (proteinuria), minimize the development and progression of kidney disease, improve polycystic kidney disease, and protect against lupus nephritis (inflammation of the kidneys caused by systemic lupus). Flaxseeds are also rich in essential fatty acids, which studies have shown reduce inflammation of the kidneys.

LEMONS AND LIMES: These citrus fruits are rich in citric acid, which research has shown prevents the development of calcium kidney stones.

PARSLEY: The high content of chlorophyll in this herb helps to oxygenate blood and alkalize pH. Parsley is a natural diuretic, promoting the flushing of toxic waste products from the kidneys and thus reducing kidney stone formation. It has also been shown to aid in fluid balance.

PEPPERMINT LEAVES: Peppermint has a relaxing effect on the muscles of the urinary system, and it also has been shown to have strong antibacterial properties. Research indicates that it is these properties that promote the clearance of bacteria in the kidney.

POTATO JUICE: Potato juice is rich in potassium citrate, which numerous studies have demonstrated prevents kidney stones by alkalinizing the urine. It is thought to work by increasing citrate excretion and improving calcium and magnesium balance. Potassium citrate is widely used as a general recommendation for kidney stone prevention.

TURMERIC: You may know it for its prominent role in Indian cuisine, but turmeric has powerful therapeutic effects. Research indicates that turmeric protects the kidneys by reducing free radicals and inflammation while increasing the level of glutathione, which promotes the clearance of toxins. In addition, curcumin, the compound that gives turmeric its yellow-orange color, has demonstrated the ability to eliminate kidney microsomal and mitochondrial lipid peroxidation. As a result, turmeric shows promise in its ability to protect against kidney damage.

WATERMELON: A water content of about 92% makes watermelon an excellent food for kidney cleansing since it supports the movement of wastes. Watermelon also has high concentrations of potassium and sodium, which help the kidneys to regulate blood pressure and fluid balance. In addition, watermelon increases nitric oxide production, which research has shown reduces the risk of kidney disease.

KIDNEY-FRIENDLY FOOD GROUPS

ANTIOXIDANT-RICH FOODS (POMEGRANATE, BLUEBERRIES): Antioxidant-rich foods are imperative for healthy kidneys. Antioxidants protect the kidneys from toxins and reduce inflammation. They are critical for the repair of kidney tissue, the safe clearance of toxins via the kidneys, and protection against further damage.

BIOFLAVONOIDS: Found in plant foods and pollen, bioflavonoids have shown protective effects against kidney stress, toxin buildup, and high blood pressure, all of which cause damage to blood vessels. Daily consumption is important.

FIBER-RICH FOODS (FRUITS, VEGETABLES, WHOLE GRAINS): Water-soluble fiber such as pectin and mucilage in these foods may counter acidosis (acidic pH) by providing a hydrogen trap in the colon. It is thought that fiber neutralizes the concentration of acid, thereby alkalinizing the pH. In addition, many high-fiber foods contain phytate, which has been shown to prevent calcium salts, both oxalate and phosphate, from crystallizing, minimizing the risk of calcium kidney stone development.

LYCOPENE-RICH FOODS (TOMATOES, WATERMELON, PARSLEY, ASPARAGUS, CABBAGE): Lycopene is a carotenoid found to be a potent antioxidant. Increased lycopene levels are known to reduce risk for cardiovascular disease and prevent DNA oxidative damage. Due to the intimate connection between cardiovascular health and kidney health, lycopene is believed to be beneficial for improving kidney health. Furthermore, a reduction in oxidative damage may protect against kidney toxicity (nephrotoxicity).

OMEGA-3 FATTY ACIDS (HEMP SEEDS, CHIA SEEDS, FLAXSEEDS, WALNUTS): Many studies have shown that omega-3 fatty acids have an anti-inflammatory effect in the body, including reducing inflammation in the kidneys. They have also been shown to inhibit kidney tumors.

PLANT-BASED PROTEIN (NUTS, SEEDS, GRAINS, GREENS, LEGUMES, AND VEGAN PROTEIN POWDERS): Protein is important in maintaining pH balance because of its role in buffering acid. The problem occurs when too much protein is consumed, especially protein high in phosphorus (animal protein), because the protein can overwhelm the body's other buffering systems. On this kidney cleanse, plant-based proteins are included instead, because proteins are vital to pH as well. Proteins provide the amino acids needed to maintain proper pH balance and thus kidney health.

From Traditional Chinese Medicine

BLACK FOODS (BLACK WALNUTS, BLACK MUSHROOMS, BLACK SESAME SEEDS, BLACK MACA): These foods are an integral part of a kidney rejuvenation plan because they reinforce kidney energy, or kidney *jing*. They are rich in vital nutrients, including minerals and antioxidants, that have been shown to promote kidney health.

KIDNEY-SHAPED FOODS (BLACK BEANS, KIDNEY BEANS): Kidney-shaped foods support the kidneys based on the idea that like form nourishes like form.

SEEDS (FLAX, PUMPKIN, SUNFLOWER): Seeds represent the beginning of new life. Since the kidneys govern fertility, seeds are seen as a kidney-nourishing food.

KIDNEY-WEAKENING FOODS

In the same way that certain foods improve kidney health, some foods do just the opposite. What makes a food or beverage detrimental to the kidneys? It's harmful if it puts strain on the kidneys' daily functions, including pH and electrolyte balance, and blood volume and pressure regulation.

That's why this cleanse eliminates all foods and beverages that cause kidney stress. I am not telling you to give them up forever, but it is necessary to stay away from them while you're on the cleanse. This will allow your kidneys to focus on repairing themselves and clearing toxins.

Note: Some of the foods listed below are more harmful to people dealing with kidney dysfunction and disease. Remember, talk to your doctor before you change your diet.

CARBONATED BEVERAGES: In a 2007 study, the National Institute of Environmental Health Sciences demonstrated a link between carbonated beverage consumption and diabetes, high blood pressure, and kidney stones, all risk factors for chronic kidney disease. In particular, cola beverages (both regular and artificially sweetened) contain high levels of phosphoric acid, which reduce citrate levels in the urine. Low citrate levels have been associated with kidney stone formation, so this mineral imbalance increases the risk of kidney stones. High levels of phosphorus have been shown to be even more detrimental to kidney function in people dealing with kidney disease.

SODIUM: Sodium, especially in refined products such as table salt, increases the amount of calcium excreted in the urine and may also increase the level of urate, triggering the formation of calcium oxalate stone. Excess sodium also increases blood pressure because it holds excess fluid in the body, leading to high blood pressure and kidney disease. We will therefore be limiting our intake of unrefined sea salt and eliminating refined table salt and sodium from processed foods.

ARTIFICIAL SWEETENERS: Artificial sweeteners like those found in diet soda have been shown to double the risk of declining kidney function. In addition, the artificial sweetener sucralose has been shown to cause enlarged and calcified kidneys.

CAFFEINE (COFFEE, BLACK TEA, CHOCOLATE, SODA): Caffeine is a natural diuretic and stimulant that increases blood pressure, stressing the kidneys. A 2002 study by the International Society of Nephrology showed that long-term caffeine consumption exacerbated chronic kidney failure in obese and diabetic rats. A 2004 study showed that caffeine consumption increased calcium excretion in urine, leading to kidney stone formation. Sorry to say, caffeine is off the list of approved foods.

ANIMAL PROTEIN: Many studies have demonstrated the relationship between a diet high in animal protein and kidney stress. These are the effects on the kidneys:

- Increase in waste product excretion: calcium, oxalates, and uric acid
- Increase in excretion of proteins in the urine (proteinuria)
- Reduction in citrate level (citrate protects against kidney stones)
- Greater risk of kidney stone formation
- Acidic pH, leading to the leaching of calcium
- Increase in level of phosphorus, which stresses the kidneys, especially in people with kidney disease
- Worsening of chronic kidney disease

ALCOHOL: Alcohol is harmful to the kidneys in various ways. First, it increases the excretion of important minerals such as calcium, magnesium, and phosphorus, thus affecting electrolyte balance. Second, the calcium, purines, oxalates, and guanosine in some types of alcohol are metabolized to uric acid, a toxic byproduct that must be filtered by the kidneys. This process acidifies the urine, resulting in the recruitment of minerals (mainly from the bones), which further stresses the kidneys and promotes the formation of kidney stones. Third, alcohol inhibits ADH (antidiuretic hormone), leading to excessive water loss and dehydration, which wreaks havoc with the removal of toxins via urine.

DAIRY: Newer research has shown that the high phosphorus content of dairy products increases the excretion of calcium in the urine. Excess phosphorus causes an imbalance of calcium, decreasing the level of calcium in the body. The level of phosphorus rises and the level of calcium drops, causing the pH to become acidic and forcing the body to recruit calcium from the bones.

FRUCTOSE SUGAR (TABLE SUGAR, HIGH-FRUCTOSE CORN SYRUP): Fructose is a monosaccharide, or simple sugar, that increases uric acid in the body. High levels of uric acid can contribute to kidney stone formation as well as kidney disease. High fructose consumption, primarily from table sugar and high-fructose corn sytup, is also associated with an increased risk of metabolic syndrome, a combination of medical disorders that is also a risk factor for developing chronic kidney disease.

CONVENTIONAL PROTEIN POWDERS: Conventional protein powders can be toxic to the kidneys and have even caused kidney failure when consumed in high amounts. Often, protein powders are made from unhealthy sources such as conventional whey and soy. Conventional whey contains growth hormones and antibiotics, and soy is almost always genetically modified and processed in hexane. Both whey and soy can lead to hormone imbalance and an acidic pH.

In addition, it is common for protein powders to contain harmful additives such as artificial sweeteners, refined sugar, caffeine, preservatives, and flavoring substances (often MSG). These additives can cause a range of health consequences including ADD, allergies, asthma, cancer, vision loss, and kidney stress. Furthermore, the testing of 15 protein powders by Consumer Reports in 2010 revealed that many had potentially toxic levels of cadmium, arsenic, lead, and mercury. For example, one protein contained arsenic and cadmium above safety limits set by United States Pharmacopoeia (USP) for drug supplements. Another product contained not only cadmium and arsenic, but also lead and mercury. These metals are known to cause damage to the kidneys, which is exacerbated by the common overusage of protein powders. For that reason, this kidney cleanse uses only organic vegan protein powders (chia, hemp, brown rice, and pea) free of any harmful additives.

CREATINE: Although creatine is among the top supplements in sports nutrition, much controversy surrounds its potential to induce kidney failure. Many small-scale trials have claimed a direct correlation between creatine and kidney damage and dysfunction, while a couple have argued against it. Research studies have suggested that creatine may be the direct cause of certain kidney ailments. One reason for the negative effects is insufficient hydration (a high level is required with creatine supplementation). Therefore, I am going to err on the side of caution by eliminating the use of creatine supplements during the kidney cleanse.

THE ELIMINATION DIET

A very important aspect of successfully cleansing the kidneys is to reduce the overall toxic load of the body. The more waste products in the blood, the harder the kidneys have to work. To minimize the workload of the kidneys, we are going to eliminate foods known to create toxic waste products. The development of toxic waste is largely due to food allergies, food intolerances, or poor digestion. This overloads the other key players in detoxification, the liver and digestive system, leaving the toxic waste to be circulated by the blood. This waste is delivered to the kidneys to be processed, stressing kidney function. We are going to eliminate the main culprits that contribute to toxic waste in the body.

Although more restrictive diets eliminate other foods such as night-shades (potatoes, tomatoes, eggplants, and peppers) and citrus, this cleanse focuses on eliminating the following three key culprits:

UNFERMENTED SOY: Soymilk, tofu, soy cheese, soy protein, texturized vegetable protein, soybean oil, edamame, soy sauce.

Note: Only unfermented soy products are eliminated; fermented soy products (such as nama shoyu, tamari, miso, and natto) are acceptable. Research indicates that when soy is unfermented its proteins are known allergens, and allergens lead to the production of toxic waste products. Unfermented soy also contains phytic acid, sometimes termed the "antinutrient" because it can block the uptake of important minerals. Fermented soy is fine in moderation. Studies have shown that the fermenting process reduces immunoreactivity (stress on the immune system) by as much as 99%, meaning that when soy is fermented it no longer creates an allergic response in the body. The fermented soy should be organic since unconventional soy is usually genetically modified.

Also remember that all soy products contain phytoestrogens that act like the hormone estrogen in the body. Be mindful and consume in moderation to prevent potential imbalances in hormones.

GLUTEN: Wheat, semolina, barley, bran, bulgur, kamut, spelt, farina, wheat flour, rye, wheat beer.

DAIRY: Yogurt, milk, cheese, cottage cheese, creamed cheese, sour cream, crème fraîche, whipped cream, ice cream.

A list of the foods that contain unfermented soy, gluten, and dairy are included in your kidney cleanse food plan, so don't worry if you don't know exactly which foods contain those products.

CHAPTER SIX

INSTRUCTIONS FOR THE KIDNEY CLEANSE

Now that you've made it this far, you'll be relieved to know that the kidney cleanse itself is straightforward. It consists of 4 days of preparation in which you begin hydrating your body and eliminating certain foods, followed by 3 days of juice feasting and therapeutic kidney teas, followed by 3 weeks on the kidney cleanse food plan. Notice I did not say "diet"?

The main goals of the cleanse are to flush the kidneys of stagnant toxic waste products, nourish them so they can work on repairing themselves, and provide therapeutic herbs to increase their capacity to cleanse blood. The secondary aim is for you to build a framework for sustaining a healthy relationship with your kidneys—and, yes, this is a relationship that requires some effort.

The kidney cleanse is designed to last 28 days. For anyone with a history of kidney stones or kidney-related illness or chronic diseases not related to the kidneys, please consult your doctor before performing this cleanse. If your doctor is on board, I suggest following the kidney cleanse for at least 6 weeks, but refer to the "Special Programs" chapter on page 123 for details about cleansing with a kidney condition.

SHOPPING LISTS

FOR THE 3-DAY JUICE FEAST (ORGANIC)

- ☐ 3 russet potatoes (6 cups or 3 pounds)
- ☐ 6 juicing oranges
- ☐ 2 bunches of cilantro (3 cups or 4 ounces)
- ☐ 3 jalapeño chile peppers
- ☐ 3 cloves of garlic
- ☐ 6 medium, green apples
- ☐ 9 limes
- ☐ 19 medium lemons
- ☐ 3 large field cucumbers (6 cups or 1½ pounds)
- ☐ 39 ribs of celery
- ☐ 3 or 4 bunches of dandelion (7½ cups)
- ☐ 1 large piece of ginger
- ☐ 3 large bunches of parsley (6 cups or 6 ounces)
- ☐ 1 watermelon (6 cups or 2 pounds)
- ☐ 1 large pineapple (6 cups or 4 pounds)
- ☐ 3 bunches of kale (9 cups)
- ☐ 24 carrots (3 pounds)
- ☐ 6 teaspoons raw and unpasteurized apple cider vinegar
- ☐ Unrefined sea salt
- ☐ Optional: Homemade vegetable broth (if store-bought, without natural flavors and canola oil)

OTHER ITEMS YOU WILL NEED

1. Juicer

You'll find many types of juicers, each with pros and cons, in stores and online. I have a masticating Breville juicer, which I find to be more affordable, more efficient, and easier to clean up than other juicers. If you have the capital and the time, I highly recommend a hydraulic press. It's the ultimate in juicers, extracting the most juice from the pulp while retaining the highest level of nutrients, but it also requires more time for juicing. See "Resources" on page 207 for recommendations.

If you are juicing at home:

Centrifugal (uses a flat cutting blade that then spins the produce at a high speed to separate the juice from the pulp)

PROS	CONS
• inexpensive • juices quickly • easy to use	• juice oxidizes more quickly (does not retain nutrients for long periods of time) • leafy greens and herbs are harder to juice • cannot juice sprouts or wheatgrass

Masticating (uses a single auger to compact and crush produce. Juice is then squeezed through a static screen; also known as slow juicer, cold press, single gear, or single auger)

PROS	CONS
• high juice yield and low pulp • juice oxidizes slower than centrifugal • can juice wheatgrass	• longer preparation time (must cut all produce) • more costly

Twin-gear (uses two interlocking gears to press produce to extract juice)

PROS	CONS
• low oxidization, juice retains its nutritional value for longer • efficiently juices leafy greens and herbs	• expensive • contains many parts, making it more difficult to put together and clean

Hydraulic press juicer (uses a vortex triturator to grind produce into a pulp that is caught in a cloth bag; bag is then pressed to extract juice)

PROS	CONS
• extremely high juice yield • does not oxidize juice. Juice retains nutritional value up to 3 days • perfect for extracting juice from leafy greens and herbs	• highest price point • difficult to clean • time consuming to use • if you are not juicing at home: find a juice bar or health food store that uses a hydraulic press juicer

2. Blender

If you want to make the creamiest soups and smoothies, you will need a multispeed blender. It makes all the difference in the world, although you can use any good blender with a powerful motor. I personally use a Vitamix, but there are other great brands as well.

3. Kidney Tea

- Dandelion tea (30 tea bags or loose leaf tea for 30 days)
- Corn silk tea (30 tea bags or loose leaf tea for 30 days)

4. Filtered Water

5. Apple Cider Vinegar

- Raw and unpasteurized, 15 ounces

6. Tools for Adjunct Therapies

- Dry skin brush made of natural bristles for dry brushing
- Castor oil and cotton flannel for castor oil packs
- Access to a sauna, ideally with infrared heat (if you have no access, you can continue to cleanse without visiting a sauna)

7. Optional but Recommended Supplements

- DHA, silymarin
- Adaptogenic herbs: astragalus, Cordyceps sinensis

8. Kidney Cleanse–Approved Foods

- See the next chapter (page 86)

Although you could start the kidney cleanse protocol on any day, I recommend starting on a Monday. This way, juice feasting will fall on the weekend. That will allow you to be in complete control of your environment and actions, leaving plenty of time for rest and focus.

In Ayurvedic medicine it is believed that the best time for juice feasting is at the turn of the seasons, specifically in spring and fall. If possible, aim to perform the cleanse during these seasons.

Finally, I recommend that you do not perform the cleanse during an acute sickness such as the flu or a cold. You want your immune system focused on clearing wastes from the kidneys, not battling a virus. In most cases, performing the cleanse while dealing with a chronic illness is highly recommended—just be sure to consult your doctor beforehand.

PREPARATION (DAYS 1-4)

Because you will be engaging in a 3-day juice feast, please closely follow the guidelines of the preparation days. I am not telling you to do this because I want to torture you, but because I have done countless juice feasts and have learned that proper preparation saves a lot of unnecessary hardship. When you are subsisting on liquids, you need all the support you can get. Do not skip this part.

DIETARY RECOMMENDATIONS

To minimize the shock of the juice feast, you will start preparing your body by eliminating the top aggravating foods and beverages. This way, your body can start rehydrating itself and processing residual toxins, a process that will reduce the changes in the body and lessen the side effects of detoxification. Remember, when you engage in a juice feast, you are increasing the rate at which toxins are removed, so you want to minimize the toxic load to maximize the benefits.

Following these steps will ensure that you actually follow through with the cleanse. Often, so many of us try to power through things so quickly that we make changes without a solid foundation. As a result, we do really well for a few days and then burn out. That is not the goal here. Please take the time to consciously follow the steps so that you set yourself up for success.

Step 1
Eliminate from your diet (or do your best to avoid) the following:

- Caffeine: coffee, non-herbal tea (black, green, oolong), soda, energy drinks
- Fried foods: doughnuts, tempura, fried meats, egg rolls, french fries, onion rings, corn dogs, chicken tenders, taquitos, samosas, hush puppies, empanadas, chimichangas
- Red meat
- Desserts made with refined sugar: cakes, brownies, candy, ice cream, pies, puddings, sugar cereals, frosting
- Pastry: croissants, Danish, éclairs, beignets, churros, funnel cakes, fritters, store-bought snack cakes, pot pies, strudel, pop tarts, turnovers

- Refined white flour: pancakes, waffles, crackers, breakfast bars, pasta, white bread

Replace with the following:

- Purified water, fresh-pressed juices and smoothies, kombucha, coconut water, herbal teas (rooibos, chamomile, fruit teas)
- Steamed, baked, sautéed, and raw foods
- Naturally sweetened desserts made with raw honey, coconut sugar, dates, figs, whole fresh fruit, coconut milk, yacon syrup, grade B or #2 maple syrup, or molasses; "raw" desserts are often a great choice
- Free-range, hormone-free eggs and poultry; wild fish
- Organic, whole-grain, and sprouted breads only, ideally homemade, bagels, English muffins, muffins, bread, pancakes, waffles (for brand name recommendations, see "Resources" on page 207)

I'll be honest, eliminating many of these foods is not going to be easy. Sugar, refined carbohydrates, and caffeine are all highly addictive substances that influence body chemistry. It is possible you will go through a period of craving these foods. It is even possible to have withdrawal symptoms such as headaches, fatigue, and anxiety. The good news is that your body will normalize as long as you push through.

Replacing these addictive substances with healthy practices such as drinking plenty of water, eating nutritious foods, and getting 30 minutes of exercise and lots of sunshine daily will help minimize any withdrawal symptoms, so do the best you can.

Step 2

Begin increasing your water intake. If you normally consume caffeinated drinks, replace all those drinks with water.

Aim to consume half your weight in ounces of filtered water daily. If you weigh 140 pounds, then drink 70 ounces of water a day. A great way to get an idea of how much you'll be drinking a day is to buy a gallon jug and fill it with your allotted water for the day. That way, you can see your goal.

The best way to make sure you reach your water goal is to be prepared. Always have a glass or BPA-free plastic water bottle with you ready to go. Typically, most of us miss out on a water opportunity when we are on the road. We start to feel thirsty, hungry, or tired (all signs of dehydration), and instead of getting water, we reach for a soda or sugary beverage. Plan ahead by filling a large water bottle before you leave the house.

Another great way to reach your water goal is to start the day with a glass filled with 16 ounces (2 cups) of room-temperature water. It's one of my favorite health tricks. First thing in the morning before you drink anything else or eat, fill a large glass (I use a Mason jar) with the water. Then add the juice of ½ lemon and 1 tablespoon of apple cider vinegar. Make sure the apple cider vinegar is raw and unpasteurized. Do your very best to drink all the water before you continue with your day or have breakfast. This not only knocks out 16 ounces of your total water goal for the day, but it also begins the natural cleansing process for the day. (Note: I recommend using a straw to prevent any damage to tooth enamel from the lemon juice.)

The room-temperature water encourages a bowel movement and kidney filtration, the apple cider vinegar stimulates digestion and promotes an alkaline pH, and the lemon juice stimulates liver detoxification and awakens the adrenal glands. This morning routine will be a part of the actual kidney cleanse, so getting used to it now, in the preparation period, gives you a jump start.

Remember, the better you do during preparation, the better you will do later on in the cleanse.

Just to be clear, the first 4 days of the cleanse are preparation days that include the following:

- Water consumption: Half your weight in ounces of filtered water daily
- Upon rising: 16 ounces (2 cups) of filtered water with the juice of ½ lemon and 1 tablespoon of apple cider vinegar
- Diet modifications: Replacing unhealthy foods with wholesome, kidney-friendly foods

THE 3-DAY JUICE FEAST (DAYS 5–7)

Once you finish the 4 days of preparation, you will dive right into the juice feast. Listed below are the guidelines for the next 3 days. I didn't list water consumption other than the 16 ounces in early morning, but try to reach your goal of half your weight in ounces of water a day. Because the juices have a high water content, you may not be as thirsty as usual.

A note about drinking juice: Swish the juice around in your mouth a few times before swallowing. This activates the salivary enzymes that stimulate the breakdown and absorption of the nutrients in the juice.

Note: Dandelion and corn silk are both natural diuretics, meaning they promote the production of urine. Don't drink these teas later than 5 p.m. to avoid having to urinate during the night.

Waking	Stick with the body's natural rhythm by waking no later than 7 a.m. This encourages you to get to bed earlier, which is extremely helpful in the cleansing process.
Upon rising	16 ounces of purified room-temperature water with the juice of ½ lemon and 1 tablespoon of apple cider vinegar
	Calming activity: Kidney yoga poses and stretches, light walk, meditation, reading
	Adjunct therapy: Dry brushing in the shower (see page 108)
Breakfast	Kidney Cleanse Juice #1 (page 137)
Midmorning	Kidney Cleanse Juice #2 (page 137)
	1 cup of kidney tea (corn silk or dandelion)
Lunch	Kidney Cleanse Juice #3 (page 138)
Afternoon	Kidney Cleanse Juice #4 (page 138)
	1 cup of kidney tea (corn silk or dandelion)
	Exercise: Kidney yoga poses and stretches, swimming, running, hiking

Dinner	Kidney Cleanse Juice #5 (page 138)
Before bedtime	Vegetable broth (only if you are hungry; try to finish within 2 hours of bedtime to avoid waking up at night to urinate)
	Stress-reduction activity: Reading, walking, playing with the dog, crafts, hot bath
	Adjunct therapy: Dry brushing in the shower (see page 108), sauna
Bedtime	Try to go to bed as early as possible. Between 9 and 10 p.m. is highly recommended to allow the body optimal time to detoxify and regenerate.

ADJUNCT THERAPIES

- Sauna: I urge you to schedule a sauna appointment during the juice feast. An infrared sauna is ideal, but if one is not accessible to you, a regular hot sauna is fine. Feel free to use the sauna every day, but even one time during the 3 days will be very helpful.

- Dry brushing: Do it once a day, during your shower. See page 108 for details.

- Colonic or enema: If you are constipated and not having a bowel movement every day, make an appointment for a colonic or perform an enema at home (see page 87 for details). It is very important to make sure your bowels are moving.

THE 3-WEEK KIDNEY CLEANSE FOOD PLAN (DAYS 8–28)

After kick-starting the cleanse with the 3-day juice feast, now you are going to gain real traction with the 3-week food plan. This is where the kidneys are given the time and the nutrient power to rebuild, restrengthen, and revitalize.

During the next 3 weeks, you will be following the kidney-supportive food plan. Each meal, snack, and beverage is part of this plan, and the more closely you follow the plan, the better your results. I am trusting that your desire to be well fosters the determination needed for follow-through.

You will find recipes for meals and snacks in the chapter starting on page 137. If you aren't able to make your own dishes, please refer to the Kidney Cleanse Shopping List on page 213 to choose the right ingredients for your meal.

Below is your daily schedule for the cleanse. I didn't list water consumption other than the 16 ounces to start the day—but, remember, consume half your weight in ounces of water daily (that includes the 16 ounces taken in the morning).

Make sure to eat dinner at least 3 hours before bedtime to avoid overburdening the digestive system and creating a toxic load in the body. If it is too late, have a light soup, kidney cleanse juice, or smoothie.

Note: If you have a history of kidney stones, every day incorporate 16 ounces of potato juice from the 3-day juice feast. See page 64 for more information about potato juice.

Upon rising	16 ounces of purified room-temperature water with the juice of ½ lemon and 1 tablespoon of apple cider vinegar
	Calming activity: Kidney yoga poses and stretches (page 97), light walk, meditation, reading
Breakfast	One smoothie option from the "Recipes" chapter (or refer to the food lists, page 213, to construct your own smoothie from kidney-supportive foods)
	Supplements (if using)
Midmorning	1 cup of kidney tea (dandelion or corn silk)
	One snack option from the "Recipes" chapter (or refer to the food lists, page 213, to construct your own snack from the kidney-supportive foods). Also a great time to drink a kidney cleanse juice
Lunch	One lunch option from the "Recipes" chapter (or refer to the food lists, page 213, to construct your own lunch from kidney-supportive foods)

Afternoon	1 cup of kidney tea (dandelion or corn silk) and a light snack (see the food lists, page 213)
	Exercise: Kidney yoga poses and stretches, swimming, running, hiking
Dinner	One dinner option from the "Recipes" chapter (or refer to the food lists, page 213, to construct your own breakfast from kidney-supportive foods)
	Supplements (if using)
After dinner	Stress-reduction activity: Reading, walking, playing with the dog, crafts, hot bath
	Adjunct therapy: Acupressure, castor oil pack, dry brushing, kidney yoga poses and stretches, sauna (for details, see page 81)
Bedtime	For optimal restoration of the organs, it's best to be in bed by 10 p.m. Aim for a minimum of 5 consecutive hours of sleep, but 7 to 8 hours are ideal.

ADJUNCT THERAPIES

- Castor oil pack: Place a castor oil pack over the kidneys for 30 minutes two to three times a week. I like doing it at the end of the day once I have time to relax, but you can do it anytime.

- Acupressure: At the end of the day when you have time to relax or are in bed, massage the K1 acupressure point (the ball of the foot between the second and third metatarsals) on the sole of one foot. Use the tip of your thumb to press and knead the point fairly deeply (but not so much that it causes excessive pain) for 1 to 2 minutes. If your thumb gets tired, rest it for a moment and then continue. Repeat with the other foot, using your other thumb. Aim to do this therapy at least four times a week, although you can do it daily if you like.

- Yoga poses and stretches: At the beginning and/or end of the day, choose a few yoga postures to promote kidney health; see a variety of recommended poses starting on page 97. Spend at least 5 minutes daily on yoga.

- Sauna: Schedule time for a once-weekly sauna. An infrared sauna is ideal but not necessary to reap benefits. A regular hot sauna will do.
- Dry brushing: Perform dry brushing daily, during your shower or at the end of the day.

For more information and instructions on the adjunct therapies, see "Lifestyle Practices While on the Cleanse" (page 86). Although these therapies are not required, they are highly recommended for optimal cleansing.

SUGGESTED SUPPLEMENTS

The juice feast and the kidney cleanse food plan are the foundation for revitalization of the kidneys, but if you want to maximize the cleansing and rebuilding process, as well as support your *jing*, then I suggest using supplements.

Supplements are an excellent way to provide additional nutrients otherwise not present in therapeutic amounts in food. Targeted nutrients have a therapeutic effect by providing the body with additional tools to heal, thereby expediting and deepening the cleansing process. This is particularly important for anyone dealing with a chronic disease or illness, because even higher amounts of nutrients are needed for function and repair.

Do you remember the discussion about adaptogenic herbs in the section on traditional Chinese medicine? Yep, this is where they come into play. Adaptogenic herbs are the most effective way to retain your *jing*, which is essential for tapping into true kidney revitalization and also for supporting the body while it undergoes detoxification. To reap the benefits of kidney *jing*, I highly recommend using the adaptogenic supplements astragalus and *Cordyceps sinensis*.

Each of the recommended supplements are live-source, meaning they come from living foods and herbs and are not made synthetically. Furthermore, they are vegan, gluten-free, and dairy-free. As confident as I am in their effectiveness, I always suggest that you discuss taking supplements with your doctor to make sure they are right for you.

CORDYCEPS SINENSIS

A fungus used in traditional Chinese medicine for nephritis (inflammation of the kidneys), *Cordyceps sinensis* is highly valued as a kidney tonic. In a host of studies, it has proved beneficial to kidney function—from improving function in people with kidney failure to protecting the kidneys from injury. It has also been shown to benefit people dealing with complicated kidney issues such as IgA nephropathy, kidney transplants, and damage due to drug and environmental toxins. Finally, *Cordyceps* is a key adaptogenic herb, promoting the preservation of kidney *jing*. I believe that it is one of the most valuable tools for improving kidney energy and health, making it one of my top recommendations for the cleanse.

Recommendation: Kidney Support by Quantum Nutrition Labs, Cordyceps or Cordyceps Munchable by Dragon Herbs

Note: Kidney Support also contains other powerful players in supporting kidney function—including asparagus, celery, and turmeric—making it one of my favorite products for the kidneys for any health status.

ASTRAGALUS (*ASTRAGALUS MEMBRANACEUS*)

Astragalus has been used in traditional Chinese medicine for thousands of years as an adaptogenic tonic herb. It contains high levels of antioxidants, which protect the body's cells—specifically in the kidneys and liver—from damage. In preliminary research studies, astragalus has demonstrated protective effects on the kidneys, especially in people with hypertensive kidney damage and diabetic nephropathy. It has also shown promise in its ability to treat kidney disease. Finally, astragalus is thought to increase blood flow in the kidneys and to reduce kidney inflammation.

Recommendation: Astragalus capsules or Astragalus eeTee by Dragon Herbs

SILYMARIN

Extracted from milk thistle, silymarin contains several potent antioxidants that have shown protective effects on kidneys. It has been shown to protect kidney cells from drug-induced nephrotoxicity (damage to the kidney from toxins), chemically induced kidney cancer, and fibrosis. In addition, in a study done on rats silymarin proved effective in protecting against ischemia (restriction of blood flow to the tissue) and reperfusion injury (tissue damage due to ischemia) in acute kidney failure. The supplement's protective effects are due to its ability to stabilize the cell membrane, act as an anti-inflammatory, and offset free radical damage.

Silymarin is also a vital nutrient for the liver because it helps to regenerate liver tissue and protect against damage, which is very important when cleansing the body.

Recommendation: Silymarin from Pure Encapsulations

Keep in mind...

When using supplements, please follow the dosages on the labels. I recommend that you take the supplements with meals, but if you are unable to or forget, you can take them in between meals.

If you are dealing with health conditions, remember to consult with your doctor prior to taking supplements.

DHA (DOCOSAHEXAENOIC ACID)

DHA is an omega-3 fatty acid found throughout the body. It is the primary structural component of the brain, skin, sperm, and retina. DHA is made from the essential fatty acid ALA (alpha linoleic acid) or obtained directly from an algae or fish source, but most people are unable to obtain adequate levels of DHA because bad fats are so pervasive in the American diet. DHA deficiency has been shown to play a role in depression, ADD, inflammation, cardiovascular disease, Alzheimer's disease, and cognitive development.

So, what does DHA have to do with the kidneys? Studies are now showing that DHA supplementation can increase the rate at which the kidneys filter waste products, reduce the excretion of protein through the urine, and improve blood movement through the kidneys. Studies have also demonstrated DHA's ability to suppress kidney injury and high blood pressure, and inhibit the development of proteinuria (the loss of blood through the urine when the glomeruli of the kidneys are damaged).

Recommendation: DHA-200 by Quantum Nutrition Labs

CHAPTER SEVEN

LIFESTYLE PRACTICES WHILE ON THE CLEANSE

During the cleanse you'll have a few other aspects of your health to address through lifestyle practices that will make the cleansing process much easier. The nice thing about these practices is that they are the tools for promoting a healthy body, even after your month on the cleanse is over. Nothing like more knowledge under your belt, right?

OPENING UP THE ELIMINATORY CHANNELS

It's important to make sure that the other eliminatory organ, the colon, is doing its job so that it is not dumping more toxins into the blood that the kidney will have to clean up. Although the proper function of the colon may not seem relevant to cleansing the kidneys, if you remember the lessons of traditional Chinese medicine, the organs are all connected. So, yes, what is happening in the colon is vital to the kidneys, especially if you want to effectively cleanse the kidneys.

If you are not eliminating toxins properly from the bowels, then those toxins may enter the bloodstream and end up in the kidneys. You better bet that we are not going to let the colon get in the way of successfully cleansing the kidneys! I am going to tell you how to give the colon a little bit of love to make sure it's on board with the master plan.

THE BASICS OF BOWEL ELIMINATION

What goes in must come out. In this case, it is called a bowel movement, and I'll share a little secret. Bowel movements should occur at least once a day, but ideally two or three times a day. Yep, you heard me all right. Up to three times a day.

The majority of us are so constipated that we think that multiple daily bowel movements indicate some kind of disease. However, multiple daily bowel movements are necessary for cleansing the body and critical for a happy and healthy body.

Now that you are wondering how in the world you got yourself into this mess, I'll give you a few basics about getting your bowels moving. If you don't get them moving, then you'll be living in a slew of toxins backing up in other places such as the kidneys. This can lead to the degradation of kidney function and makes cleansing the kidneys all the more difficult.

Since this book is not on how to cleanse the colon, I am going to give you a quick and easy rundown.

If you are not having at least one bowel movement a day, choose either the short way (an enema) or the long way (supplements and dietary tacts)—or both—to make it happen.

Enemas

Dating back to Ancient Egypt, an enema is an extremely effective yet gentle way to get the bowels moving. Although the majority of you may not even consider this an option, it is by far the best method for relieving constipation, and I think the only problem you will encounter is how much you like enemas. I know this because once you discover what it feels like to have your bowels evacuated multiple times a day, you can never go back.

The How-To

You can do an enema a day if you are really constipated, or you can do enemas a few times a week as needed. I recommend that you start with a simple warm water enema, and if you really feel inclined you can build up to a coffee enema (organic coffee beans only), which is used in holistic practices to promote detoxification, especially of the liver and gallbladder. Note: Do a coffee enema only under the guidance of a licensed practitioner.

Enema buckets can be found at most pharmacies or can be ordered online. Make sure to follow the directions carefully. While an enema is not difficult to do yourself, you will want to perform it correctly to prevent any complications. It is a good idea to consult your doctor first, especially if you are dealing with any issues of the bowels, anus, or cardiovascular system.

A Word About Colonics

For many of you, the concept of administering your own enema is more than you can handle, so using a colon hydrotherapist and colon irrigation systems may be your best option. Colon hydrotherapists (the practitioners who administer colonics) believe that colonics are more effective than enemas since they are able to draw out stagnant waste that enemas cannot reach. On the other hand, some people speculate that colonics may sometimes cause intestinal complications. I recommend that you talk with your doctor before undergoing colon irrigation, and always go to a licensed hydrotherapist.

Supplements and Diet-Specific Tactics

If you are following the kidney cleanse food plan as well as the guideline to drink half your weight in ounces of water daily and you are still not having a daily bowel movement after 1 week, then it may be necessary for you to use supplements. Supplements often get to the root cause of constipation, while enemas help bridge the gap until you can have a bowel movement on your own.

Many factors contribute to constipation, but the five basic things a person must consume daily for proper elimination are sufficient water, unrefined sea salt, fiber, healthy oil/fat, and probiotics. The good news is that all those bases are covered in the kidney cleanse, so they shouldn't be a cause of your continued constipation other than perhaps probiotics.

Probiotics are healthy bacteria in your intestines that are vital for proper digestion as well as for a healthy immune system and even emotional balance. You can usually maintain a proper balance of healthy bacteria in the gut by eating foods rich in probiotics, unless you have a history of antibiotic use, a bowel condition, or a history of eating junk foods. These conditions could deplete the healthy bacteria to the point that supplementation is necessary.

How do antibiotics affect probiotics?

Antibiotics are substances designed to kill microorganisms (the word "antibiotic" means "anti-life"). When used to treat bacterial infections, they kill or inhibit the growth of good bacteria, like probiotics, along with bad bacteria. If you have taken antibiotics, you most likely are suffering from inadequate levels of healthy bacteria in the gut, which may be a root cause of your constipation. Supplementing with a probiotic will help restore the healthy bacteria.

You may wonder why you cannot simply increase your consumption of probiotic-rich foods such as organic kefir, yogurt, sauerkraut, or kombucha. The problem is that often the healthy bacteria in the gut have been so depleted that probiotic-rich foods alone may not restore them. A probiotic supplement is often a necessary route to fully repopulate the gut and restore normal bowel movements.

Recommendation: Probiotic by Quantum Nutrition Labs or Dr. Ohhira's

Other Root Causes of Constipation

If your gut is housing a healthy population of probiotics, then your constipation may be due to one of the other main root causes of constipation: poor digestion or adrenal stress that results in a magnesium deficiency.

The Digestion Connection

Earlier I said that what goes in must come out. There's an exception: when the body can't break down the food that was consumed. When the body is fed certain foods, especially processed, high-protein, and mucus-forming foods, most often it cannot properly digest them. As a result, the foods rot and often form mucus in the gut, which prevents healthy stools from forming, leading to constipation.

Although you may be thinking that this cannot be an underlying issue for you since you are consuming only healthy foods, in some cases the body is unable to break down even healthy foods. A history of eating unhealthy foods can also cause congestion in the colon. The basics of uncovering the root of constipation begins with proper digestion.

When addressing the health of the digestive system and proper bowel movements, it is vital to examine diet—but on the kidney cleanse food plan, this isn't a relevant factor. The next step is to provide the body with basic supplements to promote proper digestion and elimination. The two most elementary supplements that support healthy digestion and elimination are the following:

- HCl (hydrochloric acid): To supplement gastric acid produced by the stomach
- Digestive enzymes: To supplement enzymes produced by the stomach, pancreas, and small intestine

The supplementation of both HCl and digestive enzymes is the best way to address constipation. For many people, these digestive aids do the trick. In the rare case that they don't provide relief, you may have to look further—to magnesium supplementation.

Recommendation: Betaine HCl and Digest by Quantum Nutrition Labs

The Magnesium-Constipation Connection

Magnesium has been used clinically for its laxative effect, and thus its supplementation is recommended for cases of constipation that are not resolved by digestive supplements. Magnesium causes water to be retained in the intestines, which promotes the fluidity of the bowels, resulting in a bowel movement and constipation relief.

But why are we talking about magnesium? Because magnesium deficiency is a common problem and is worth exploring as an underlying factor in stubborn cases of constipation.

How does a person become magnesium deficient? Magnesium is expended at high levels when the body is under stress. This occurs because stress causes the adrenal glands to release adrenaline. In turn, the adrenals call for the release of magnesium, which has a calming effect on the body. Because most of us are constantly stressed, our bodies are continuously dealing with the overproduction of adrenaline, which depletes magnesium. But stress is not the only reason for chronic magnesium deficiency. Other factors include excessive exercise, heavy sweating, an imbalanced diet, high sugar intake, and alcohol or caffeine use. If you are chronically fatigued or stressed, magnesium supplementation may be the answer to stubborn constipation, especially if you are abiding by the five basic rules of a healthy bowel movement: sufficient water, unrefined sea salt, fiber, healthy fat, and probiotics.

Recommendation: Magnesium Glycinate by Pure Encapsulations

I hope that by now you are fully aware of the importance of pH to kidney health and understand why I keep talking to you about alkalizing your pH. If you are working on alkalizing your pH and the goal is to get your pH in range, how will you know if you are there?

You will know by tracking your pH with urinary pH test strips. The great part about tracking the pH of your urine is that you have direct feedback on the potential toxic burden of your kidneys. The kidneys are in charge of pH balance, so when pH is not in the ideal alkaline range, there's reason to believe the kidneys are under stress. It's important to know your pH while on the cleanse because that will tell you if you need to modify your practices, such as increasing your consumption of green vegetables or unrefined sea salt. Make sense?

Recommendation: Purchase urinalysis test strips and measure your pH every morning. You will have to measure your first morning urine since this is most indicative of the true pH. Ideally, the pH of your first morning urine should be 6.5 to 7.0. Throughout the day your pH should become more alkaline, reaching a range of 7.5 to 8.0 by the evening.

HOW TO READ YOUR PH

If the pH of your urine is below 6.5, your body is in an acidic state. This means that there is more acid being created than your body can buffer with its mineral reserves. We can assume that the kidneys are under more stress since they have to filter the acidic ash residue. (Do you remember the concept of ash residue based on Dr. Robert Young's *The pH Miracle?*) In addition, an acidic pH indicates that you are losing minerals, which can lead to bone loss down the line.

If the pH of your urine is 8.0 or higher, you are in a extreme alkaline state — which, though seemingly contradictory, indicates a state of severe acidity. When the body becomes so acidic that it loses its alkaline reserves (minerals needed to buffer the acid), ammonia and bicarbonate are excreted through the urine, causing the pH to be extremely alkaline. This often occurs in people who consume too much protein, because ammonia typically converts to urea, which is then excreted by the kidneys. It is the ammonia that is causing the alkaline pH, which actually indicates a severe degree of acidosis (acidic pH). This situation is undesirable because the mineral deficit stresses the kidneys.

A healthy pH balance is controlled not only by diet but also by a well-functioning digestive system. If your body is not properly digesting food, then the mineral content is not in a form that can be readily accepted by the cells. If the cells cannot use the minerals, then the body cannot properly balance pH. Often, hydrochloric acid (HCl) and digestive enzymes are needed to improve the digestive process and make the minerals accessible. So, if your pH is out of range when you track it during the cleanse, I recommend that you increase your consumption of alkaline foods in addition to supplementing with HCl and digestive enzymes.

HOW THE KIDNEY CLEANSE AFFECTS URINE PH

The kidney cleanse promotes an alkaline pH through foods as well as through improvement of kidney function. If you record your urine pH at the beginning and end of the cleanse, you should see the pH improve to between 6.5 and 7.0. If you are testing your first morning urine pH daily and see no improvement, then one of these two situations may be occurring:

1. You are not properly digesting your food, and the use of HCl and digestive enzymes are needed.

2. You are building up your mineral (alkaline) reserves and have not accumulated enough minerals to alkalinize the pH. In this case, continue eating a good diet and supporting the kidneys and digestive system until your pH rises. This condition is common in people whose mineral reserves are depleted because they've had a bad diet for a long time.

EXERCISING

Whether you regularly exercise or hate the thought of working out, there's no getting away from it—aerobic exercise must be incorporated as a lifestyle practice on the kidney cleanse.

You may be thinking that I've added exercise to the kidney cleanse as an optional, it's-good-for-you practice, but the truth is that exercise induces profound changes in the kidneys. I didn't choose the word "profound." It comes directly from a study conducted by researchers in sports medicine. The research demonstrated that exercise makes a difference in how the kidneys excrete protein and filter toxins. Remember, the more efficiently the kidneys filter, the more successful you will be in clearing toxins during the cleanse.

The effects of exercise on people with kidney conditions

Exercise is critical in increasing the capacity of the kidneys to filter toxins, but researchers have also shown that it can be an invaluable tool for people dealing with specific kidney conditions. Let's check it out!

Kidney stones: A study conducted by Mathew Sorensen, MD, at the University of Washington School of Medicine in Seattle revealed that people who exercised had a 13% lower risk of developing kidney stones.

Chronic kidney disease: Studies indicate that exercise improves quality of life and nutrition, reduces inflammation and depression, and decreases treatment costs and the need for hospitalization. In addition, preliminary evidence, although mixed, suggests that aerobic exercise can improve blood pressure, lipid profiles, and mental outlook.

Dialysis: For those on dialysis, exercise has been found to be especially beneficial for kidney health. The recommendation is for low-intensity, non-weight-bearing exercise 3 days a week for 30 to 40 minutes.

Diabetic nephropathy: Research indicates that low-level exercise is beneficial to those with diabetic nephropathy. Independent of improvements of overweight and hyperglycemia, exercise hinders its progression while improving inflammation levels and oxidative damage, and without causing stress to the kidney.

High blood pressure: Many studies now show that regular exercise can lower blood pressure, producing sustained decreases in both systolic and diastolic pressures. Furthermore, it can even lower the level of catecholamine, a substance that increases blood pressure.

Cardiovascular health: Exercise has been shown to improve cardiovascular health including heart disease by increasing heart functioning and circulation. Improvement in cardiovascular health means improvement in kidney health since the two are intimately tied.

Although some older research indicated that exercise stresses the kidneys, newer research shows that moderate-intensity exercise is not associated with an increase in the risk of kidney damage. In fact, studies indicate that exercise doubles the kidneys' ability to filter, which is just what is needed during a kidney cleanse. In addition, aerobic exercises induce sweating, a natural way for the body to rid itself of toxins. The more toxins you can eliminate, the better!

Note: Not all forms of exercise are beneficial for the kidneys. A 2010 study revealed that marathon running can cause acute kidney injury and changes in kidney filtration—as if the pain of actually running a marathon weren't enough!

EASTERN EXERCISE PRACTICES: THE POWER OF YOGA

The practice of yoga, which dates back 5,000 years, integrates mind, body, and spirit. The goal is to take control of the body in order to quiet the mind so that a state of enlightenment is achieved. If you think that this practice is for New Age hippies and Buddhist monks, know that yoga is far more accessible than ever before. Keep an open mind and see how yoga can benefit your cleansing.

What Does Yoga Have to Do with Cleansing the Kidneys?

A lot, actually. Yoga has far-reaching effects on the kidneys, making it an extremely beneficial therapy during the cleansing process. Yoga has the ability to influence the kidneys in the following four ways:

1. Opening the Kidney Meridian

The body is made up of meridians, or channels, that serve as highways for the transfer of energy throughout the body. Yoga can open these pathways, allowing the life energy, or qi, to flow. Each body system is fed by a meridian in much the same way that the circulatory system carries blood. It is through the transfer of this energy that vitality and balance is brought to the organs and glands and to the balancing energies, yin and yang. It is through these pathways that communication throughout the body is synced.

Just as highways become congested with traffic, so can the meridians. When meridians are congested, energy is obstructed or blocked, leading to dysfunction of organs or gland systems. When the kidney meridian is blocked, the kidneys can't properly clear toxins or receive nutrients—and you can't properly detoxify. Using targeted yoga poses and postures will open up the kidney meridians. Once these channels are open, the kidneys will be able to receive the nutrients they need to eliminate any toxins. Pretty cool, huh?

2. Physically Manipulating the Tissue

Ever feel lower back pain or stiffness? This often happens when the fascia, or band of fibrous tissue, around the kidneys becomes restricted. This physical tightness can occur due to surgical scars, adhesions, lack of stretching, poor posture, or injury. The tightness interferes with kidney function. Using targeted yoga stretches to make sure the fascia around the kidneys is mobile and flexible is a great way to improve kidney circulation, blood and lymphatic flow, and nerve supply. Regular yoga practice also promotes proper spinal alignment and posture, relieving stress on the lower back and kidneys.

Another possible benefit of yoga is its ability to break up fibrin deposits in the kidneys. Fibrin is a fibrous protein that creates deposits due to a variety of events such as cell and tissue degradation and persistent inflammation. This leads to a type of scarring that inhibits normal kidney functioning. As a result, utilizing yoga as a means of breaking up fibrin deposits may be an important avenue to explore, especially for those with kidney disease, since there are limited treatments for this condition.

3. Promoting a Parasympathetic (Kidney-Healing) State

Another benefit of yoga is its role in sympathetic and parasympathetic dominance. The sympathetic and parasympathetic systems make up the autonomic nervous system, which controls unconscious and conscious body functions, including heart rate, perspiration, urination, and even breathing.

The sympathetic nervous system promotes the "fight or flight" response, preparing the body for attack. This includes generating energy, increasing heart rate, and inhibiting digestion, and all catabolic activities (activities that break the body down). The parasympathetic nervous system promotes the "rest and digest" response. This system is concerned with nourishing, healing, regenerating the body, and all anabolic activities (activities that build the body up). These activities include digestion, urination, and defecation.

A fine balance between these two systems is vital to human health, because when imbalance occurs, especially when the sympathetic system dominates, the body becomes more susceptible to disease. Your goal is to remain predominantly in a parasympathetic state so that your body can focus on healing and detoxifying. Make sense?

Releasing tension in the soft tissues is thought to promote a parasympathetic state in the body. All soft tissues are innervated by the sympathetic nervous system, and when they are stressed through tension or poor posture, the sympathetic nervous system dominates. By using yoga as a form of exercise, you will be able to promote a parasympathetic state, necessary for the proper cleansing and rejuvenation of the kidneys.

4. Quieting the Mind and Reducing Stress

Yoga is acclaimed for its ability to make you as limber as Gumby and for its mind-clearing, stress-reducing effects on the body, leaving you humming in a Zenlike state for hours. How exactly does the practice of yoga and the absence of stress improve the effects of a kidney cleanse?

The physical postures of yoga quiet the mind in much the same way that they put your body into a parasympathetic state. The body responds not just to physical movements, but also to internal messages sent by the mind. It is as important to address the body physically as it is to address it mentally, and fortunately yoga does both.

When the body is stressed physically, mentally, or spiritually, it sends a message to the adrenal glands to jump into gear and release "fight or flight" hormones. This launches the body into a sympathetic state. As a result, the kidneys become stressed as they strive to balance the cascade of reactions created by the adrenals. In the sympathetic state, especially if it is chronic, the kidneys are unable to focus on clearing toxins, let alone regenerate tissue. It is imperative to keep stress levels down by using the mind-clearing techniques of yoga so that the kidneys can focus on cleansing instead of reacting to the adrenals on hyper drive.

Yoga Targeted for the Kidneys

Now that you are more convinced than ever that you need to start practicing yoga, I have put together a sequence of poses targeting the kidneys. Your goal is to practice these poses at least once a day while on the cleanse. Don't worry, you can do them all in under 10 minutes. They get your body moving and your energy flowing, which should feel good.

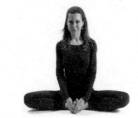

Butterfly Pose

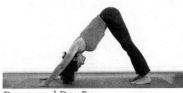

Downward Dog Pose

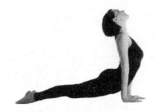

Upward Dog Pose

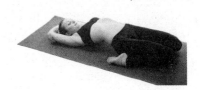

Saddle Pose

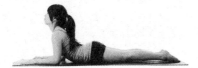

Sphinx Pose

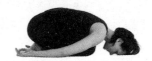

Child's Pose

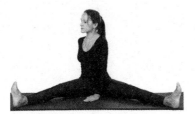

Straddle Pose

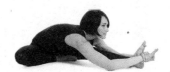

Knee-to-Head Forward Fold Pose
(Janu Sirsasana)

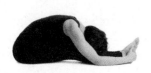

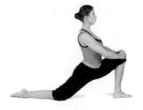

Full Forward Pose (Paschimottanasana)   The Hurdler or Runner's Stretch

The Iliopsoas-Kidney Connection

One final pose of prime importance to kidney health is the hurdler or runner's stretch. This pose is incredibly important because of its ability to open up the iliopsoas, among the most significant muscles in the body. Running down the back of the spine and connecting at the front of the thighbone, it plays a crucial role in general body support. Its location is significant because when it becomes tight it shortens. The result is a swayback, with the pelvis tilting forward and the butt pushing out. A structural imbalance like this stresses the organs. A tight, contracted iliopsoas causes a biomechanical imbalance in the posture and can result in the kidneys being compressed. Making sure the iliopsoas is loose and pliable is vital for kidney health

PUTTING IT ALL TOGETHER

As you can see, whether you have healthy kidneys or a pair that need some love, exercise is an integral part of the cleansing process. I recommend exercising 3 to 6 days a week, with each session at least 20 minutes long (10 minutes of that dedicated to the yoga and stretch routine). Whether you go for a walk, join a sports team, or drag a friend to a paddle boarding lesson, find a form of exercise that works for you and that you can stick with, because committing yourself to climbing the stair stepper at the gym is not the only way to exercise. There are many more options.

REDUCING STRESS: THE MISSING LINK

If you happen to be among the 1% who live in a perfect world where stress does not exist, give me a call because I am getting a one-way ticket there. For the rest of us, all we can do is manage stress by learning how to reduce it and minimize its physiological effects on the body. Stress is a major factor in the deterioration of health, and our kidneys do not escape its wrath. Properly managing stress by integrating various strategies is essential when cleansing the kidneys.

HOW DOES STRESS AFFECT THE BODY GENERALLY?

The effects of both acute and chronic stress are far-reaching in the alteration of normal physiological processes, making stress a risk factor for a host of diseases. The following is a list of its most pronounced effects:

- Suppressed immune system
- Prolonged healing times
- Heightened vulnerability to infection
- Impaired cognition
- Decreased thyroid function
- Accumulation of abdominal fat

How exactly does stress affect your kidneys, you may wonder? To grasp the connection between stress and the kidneys, let's consider the adrenal glands.

Adrenal Glands

Did you know that the adrenal glands sit right on top of the kidneys? Their location is no coincidence. The adrenal glands and the kidneys work together, and so we cannot properly talk about kidney cleansing without addressing the adrenal glands and what happens when they're fatigued or stressed.

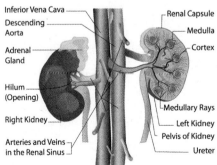

Adrenal and Kidneys

In traditional Chinese medicine, an organ is viewed as a functional system rather than as just the organ itself. The kidney system includes the kidneys, the adrenal glands, and the urinary system, all of which make up the kidney life force. A problem with the adrenal glands is often addressed by looking at the kidneys. Our interest in the adrenal glands lies in their ability to alter kidney function, a common occurrence in the case of adrenal fatigue or other forms of adrenal insufficiency or disease. In fact, adrenal fatigue is viewed as kidney deficiency in Chinese medicine.

What Is Adrenal Fatigue?

Adrenal fatigue is not necessarily a diagnosable condition by the standards of Western medicine, but its prevalence has increased interest among alternative practitioners, making it a recognizable ailment. The theory is that when the adrenal glands enter a state of chronic stress, they are unable to perform correctly, resulting in their inability to produce adequate hormones, especially cortisol. Common symptoms include extreme fatigue, inability to fall asleep, sugar and carbohydrate cravings, depression, poor memory, and a low sex drive. Improperly functioning adrenals in turn affect kidney function.

What Do the Adrenal Glands Do?

The adrenal glands are composed of two parts: the outer zone, called the adrenal cortex, and the inner zone, called the adrenal medulla. Both are vital to overall health, but the cortex is the part that's of particular interest to kidney function. It secretes steroid hormones, and the one that we are interested in is aldosterone, which acts directly on the kidneys. We talked about aldosterone earlier, in the chapter "The Kidneys and Their Role in Health" (page 18). It helps maintain blood volume and pressure by promoting sodium retention and potassium excretion.

What Happens to Aldosterone When the Adrenals Are Stressed or Not Functioning Properly?

As a response to poor adrenal function, the level of aldosterone decreases, which can lead to adverse effects on the kidneys. Insufficient production of aldosterone can lead to low blood pressure and improper sodium levels, both of which cause kidney stress and dysfunction. In fact, there has been emerging evidence implicating aldosterone involvement in the progression of kidney disease. You can see that making sure the adrenals produce enough aldosterone is vital to kidney health.

The Other Vital Hormone, Cortisol

The main function of cortisol, which is secreted by the adrenal cortex, is to restore equilibrium after exposure to stress. Cortisol influences processes that affect the entire body, but let's focus on its effects on the kidneys.

The following are a few ways that cortisol affects kidney function:

- Balances the level of calcium by decreasing intestinal calcium absorption and increasing calcium excretion by the kidneys, and also by causing the breakdown of calcified bone
- Maintains normal blood pressure
- Increases glomerular filtration rate (GFR) and kidney blood flow

Obviously, having the adrenals produce enough cortisol is very important to the health of your kidneys.

The Role of Catecholamine Hormones

The adrenal medulla, the inner part of the adrenal gland, secretes catecholamines to help the body deal with physical and emotional stress. The ones we're interested in are epinephrine (adrenaline) and norepinephrine (noradrenaline).

Epinephrine, a "fight or flight" hormone, increases heart and respiratory rate, vasoconstriction and vasodilation, muscle contraction, and the breakdown of glycogen and lipids. Norepinephrine directly increases heart rate, triggering the release of glucose from energy stores and increasing blood flow to muscles.

Did you notice the words "vasoconstriction" and "vasodilation"? These hormones cause the constriction of blood vessels in the kidneys, which essentially slows down the kidneys' filtration rate.

Do you remember why it's so important to increase the kidneys' filtration rate? With an increased ability to filter, the kidneys can process more harmful toxins for excretion. If these hormones are not functioning properly, and especially if their levels are chronically high, your kidneys will be unable to filter efficiently—and if they cannot filter efficiently, how can they get rid of toxins? You can start to see the impact of adrenal hormones on the process of cleansing the kidneys.

Two other ways in which catecholamines influence the kidneys is through mineral balance and blood pressure. They reduce kidney sodium excretion, which can lead to water retention, and water retention combined with vasoconstriction can translate to high blood pressure. High blood pressure causes significant stress on the kidneys, so maintaining adrenal health is key.

Still paying attention? The point is that our goal is to minimize the "fight or flight" adrenaline response so that these adrenal hormones do not interfere with optimal functioning of the kidneys, which is vital to the process of cleansing. The good thing is that the kidney cleanse protocol calls for addressing many factors that improve adrenal health. As I mentioned at the beginning of our journey together, this cleanse is far more than just a kidney cleanse—it's a foundation for lifelong health.

TOOLS FOR REDUCING STRESS

So now that it has become blatantly clear that you must reduce stress to save your kidneys, what is the best way to do it?

You're eliminating the foods that cause stress, and you have a yoga and exercise routine. What other ways can you quiet your mind and body so that the adrenal glands can go on holiday?

The following is a list of other techniques for reducing stress. Although this may seem like a lengthy list of things to do for the cleanse, it's a great time to try something new! Pick one, pick two, or pick them all. Adding these techniques to your daily schedule, for even as little as 5 minutes a day, will result in health changes that you can actually see.

- Meditation
- Tai chi
- Reading (no celebrity gossip magazines, please)
- Calming music (jazz, classical, spa)
- Massage
- Nature walks
- Playing with your pet

- Turning off the TV!
- Taking a electronic device vacation (no iPad, computer, iPhone)
- Saying no to social media
- 5 minutes of quiet time (morning and/or night)
- Painting, drawing, sculpting, or other art
- Breathing deeply for 10 full breaths

SLEEP AND SLEEP POSITION

We all know that sleep is one of the basic tenets of good health, but how important is it during the kidney cleanse?

Sleep could be described as a barometer of health. Although sleep was once thought of as a time when the brain descended into a comalike state, it is now recognized as a process that induces a dynamic cascade of action integral to the overall health of the mind and body. It is during this time that the body can catch up on functions that it was unable to attend to because of the stressors of an awakened state.

The process of cleansing the body requires energy, and during the day that energy is often used elsewhere for functions such as digestion. Your body uses the time when you are asleep for focusing on tasks such as neutralizing and processing toxins, and regenerating tissues. This is especially important for the kidneys, because one of its main functions is to detoxify.

But that is not all! Many studies have shown that inadequate sleep has an adverse effect on the cardiovascular and endocrine (hormone) systems. This is key because these two systems greatly influence the kidneys. If your blood pressure or hormones, especially the stress and fluid/electrolyte balancing hormones, are out of range and not functioning properly, then the kidneys are burdened. Getting adequate hours of undisturbed sleep is essential during this kidney cleanse.

An interesting study showed a strong correlation between disrupted biological rhythms (due to sleep deprivation, shift work, and jet lag), and increased risk for cardiovascular and kidney disease. The researchers concluded that the renewal of organ tissues likely occurs during sleep, suggesting that sleep disruption prevents this process from happening and results in damage to the organs. One more reason to pull up the covers early!

LISTENING TO YOUR BODY, SLEEPING THROUGH THE CLEANSING PROCESS

Allowing yourself to sleep for longer hours than usual during the cleansing process will help you physically and mentally. Clearing toxins from your body can make you feel fatigued. This is normal, and I urge you to listen to your body. Give yourself permission to take it easy, get to bed early (I mean between 9 and 10 p.m.), and even nap during the day, especially during the 3-day juice feast. It is during the feast that you will find that the more you sleep, the easier it is to get through the feast and the better you feel.

Finally, allowing for more rest will help you stabilize your emotions. This is important because often a cleanse or a new health practice can make you feel out of balance or anxious and increase the danger of not following through. The more you can do to ensure success, the better. We all know that we can become unsettled when caffeine, chocolate, and alcohol are taken away, so do yourself a favor, take my advice, and plan to sleep... a lot.

CASTOR OIL

There cannot be a book about cleansing the kidneys without a discussion of castor oil packs. You may have heard of castor oil as a powerful laxative, but I am referring to its external use, not its internal use.

Castor oil comes from the castor seed, *Ricinus communis*, native to India. Its therapeutic use dates back to the ancient world, where it was called *palma christi* since the leaves were said to resemble the hand of Christ and its healing capabilities were revered as godlike. While its clinical therapeutic uses range from relieving arthritis and dermatitis to reducing the spread of tumors, we are interested in its proposed ability to stimulate the immune and lymphatic systems.

The external use of castor oil to increase lymphocyte production was first popularized by the physic healer Edgar Cayce and later by Dr. William McGarey, founder of A.R.E. Clinic in Arizona. Lymphocytes are disease-fighting white blood cells that inhabit the lymphatic system. They have a very important role in the immune system, identifying and dealing with harmful foreign substances or particles such as bacteria and other infectious organisms and toxins. If the lymphatic system becomes congested, which is common when detoxifying the body, the waste products and toxins build up and can't properly be eliminated, leading to a host of issues such as inflammation, poor toxin clearance, a depressed immune system, and disease. During the cleanse, it is very important to make sure your lymphatic system is moving properly, since cleansing pushes even more toxins through the system.

Sleep position for kidney stones

If you are a victim of kidney stones, listen up. A couple of studies suggest that sleeping position plays a role in recurrent stone formation in people with same-sided stones. The culprit is believed to be sluggish blood flow, which allows for the crystals to settle on the side you are sleeping on. If you suffer from multiple stones in the left kidney, it is highly probable that it is from sleeping on your left side, and the same for the right kidney. A simple change of position may reduce recurrence.

This is where castor oil proves useful. It is thought that the oil from an external pack will penetrate the skin, increasing lymphocyte count and sending a signal to the immune system to ramp up its identification and clearance of toxins. Therefore, we will be placing the castor oil packs over the kidneys to promote lymphatic drainage and improve the detoxification process.

In my own personal experience with castor oil packs, I have found them to be a must-have for any cleansing or rejuvenating program when used just two or three times a week, although they can be used more often. I have seen them make a difference in advancing the cleansing process and in reducing any possible side effects of cleansing. If you are dealing with any inflammation, pain, or stagnation in the area of the kidneys, I believe that they can help bring relief. Although the scientific evidence is not strong, with only one clinical study on the use of castor oil for the stimulation of the lymphatic system, clinical and anecdotal experience is much more conclusive, making it a worthwhile adjunct therapy for the kidney cleansing process.

Note: If you are dealing with a chronic disease or disorder, consult your doctor before using this treatment.

HOW TO USE CASTOR OIL PACKS

First, I want to say something about quality. Castor oil comes in a range of quality, just as olive oil does. Purchase a reputable brand (I list my favorite brands in "Resources," page 207), because castor oil manufacturers commonly use toxic solvents (hexane), pesticides, and deodorants that not only contaminate the oil but also may damage their healing properties.

You will need the following:
- Cotton flannel (organic cotton cloth)
- Plastic wrap (I like Glad Press 'n Seal)
- Cold-pressed, solvent-free castor oil
- Heating pad

Directions:
1. Cut the flannel into a triple-layer rectangle, enough to cover your lower back from hip to hip (the area of the kidneys).

2. Cut the plastic wrap so it is about 2 inches larger than the flannel on each side. (It will stick to the skin around the flannel to prevent the castor oil from spilling.)

3. Place the flannel on the plastic wrap and saturate it with about 3 to 4 tablespoons of castor oil. The flannel should be wet, but not dripping.

4. Find a comfortable place to sit (couch, bed, or chair) where you will remain for the next 30 minutes to an hour. If you are sensitive, start with a 15-minute session to make sure you do not react adversely. Plug in the heating pad nearby so you can access it while seated.

5. Place the cloth and plastic wrap over the kidneys (lower back from hip to hip). Then cover with the heating pad. Make sure the wrap is hot enough to feel, but not hot enough to be uncomfortable.

6. Sit back and relax. Take this time to read, listen to music, or enjoy a conversation.

7. Once finished, wash off with nontoxic soap and water.

Note: Make sure that castor oil does not get on your clothing or furniture because it may stain.

ACUPRESSURE

You have already learned about the importance of opening the kidney meridian through the use of targeted yoga poses and postures, but there is another avenue to reach this goal: acupressure. Acupressure is similar to acupuncture, but without those dreaded needles (yes, I am a proclaimed sissy). The use of acupressure to open meridians to increase the flow of chi or energy has been pretty well received by the holistic community and has shown its effectiveness in many studies.

Although there are many kidney points used in acupressure, we are only going to focus on K1, which is found at the bottom of the foot. K1 is a major energy vortex with the ability to revitalize body, mind, and spirit, making it a perfect point for the kidney cleanse. This point is often used to ground a person's energy, especially when the person is obsessing or feeling anxious about things, as we all often are. Furthermore, it is a common point used for helping high blood pressure, insomnia, and headaches.

HOW TO PERFORM ACUPRESSURE

1. Find the K1 point on the sole of the foot between the second and third metatarsal bones.

2. Using your thumb, apply even pressure to the point.

3. Hold firmly or slightly massage for about 1 minute.

If this point is tender, perform for a shorter time or use less pressure.

DRY BRUSHING

Dry brushing uses a brush made of natural bristles to remove the top layer of dead skin. The theory, although unproven in scientific studies, is that removal of dead skin cells opens the pores and promotes the elimination of toxins. Dry brushing is also thought to stimulate the lymphatic system to more efficiently transfer nutrients and remove waste at a cellular level. By increasing the elimination of toxins, you can theoretically reduce the toxic load to the kidneys and increase the effectiveness of the cleanse.

Although the practice of dry brushing does not have a strong scientific foundation, it is a widely accepted detoxification technique used by holistic practitioners as an effective adjunct to cleansing programs. Besides, no one ever complained of having softer and more supple skin, which dry brushing most certainly accomplishes!

HOW TO DRY BRUSH

1. Begin dry brushing after the skin has warmed in a hot shower or bath.

2. Start with your feet and, using circular movements, brush toward your heart.

3. Continue up each leg until you reach the top of the thigh and buttock.

4. Next continue up each arm, beginning at the fingertips and working toward the heart. Once you reach the shoulders, stop.

5. Next move to your torso, beginning at the back and then moving to your stomach. Once you get to your stomach, work up to your heart and finish there.

6. Rinse and shower as normal.

CHAPTER EIGHT

AFTER THE CLEANSE

Congratulations! You made it! You successfully accomplished the cleanse. Are you wondering what to do next?

I wish I could tell you it's okay to go back to fast food, caffeine, or hard partying, but if you really want to maintain your health, especially your kidney health, then you must consider some permanent lifestyle changes. Now, don't let the word "permanent" scare you off.

Realize that your body is on a roll right now, making your follow-through just as important as the cleanse itself. If you are truly interested in radiant health, you will want to follow through, because the reintroduction of bad habits has that annoying ability to destroy all your hard work. So, while you are officially at the "end" of the kidney cleanse, you are actually at a crossroads. Choose the road that ensures permanent health changes!

PRISTINE BODY, CLEAN KIDNEYS: KEEPING THE BALL ROLLING

Imagine this: Your body has just undergone a radical spa month at the top retreat in Palm Springs, California, and you were there so long that your body forgot what cheese, steak, and wine were. It finally started to function well, having cleared up nagging problems and regained youthful energy. Just as you wouldn't want to throw yourself into a pile of freezing snow after an hour in a hot tub, you do not want to shock your newly cleansed body with toxic foods and lifestyle practices. It's now time to make your way back into the "real" world, where happy hour may be an option on your social calendar and a cream cheese bagel may be on the menu.

STEP 1: REINTRODUCING FOODS

As I'm sure you remember clearly, a lot of foods were eliminated during the kidney cleanse. The question is, do you dive right back in or do you reintroduce foods slowly?

The answer is to reintroduce them slowly. While I encourage you to keep following the kidney cleanse food plan (it delivers a powerhouse of nutrients), I realize that this is just not in the cards for many of you. Thus, the goal is to reintroduce the foods groups one by one so you can identify any possible and lingering food intolerances.

This concept comes from the elimination diet, a tool for identifying food allergies. The diet eliminates food groups that commonly cause allergic responses and then reintroduces them one at a time. That way, a person can monitor how he or she feels and recognize any adverse effects the foods may have. I am a huge fan of this concept and find it to be extremely helpful in identifying which foods work for the body and which do not, because we all react to and require different foods. Use this precious time when your body is clean and pure to flag the bad guys that may have been the root cause of your kidney issues and even a chronic ailment, such as inflammation, psoriasis, or headaches.

Note: It is possible that some of your previous food intolerances have now cleared, making those foods okay to eat again. This is because your body has had time to detoxify, releasing the "memory" of the toxin from the immune system, as well as time to heal the intestinal lining.

The Reintroduction Plan

The strategy is to reintroduce food groups one at a time. Every 3 days you will reintroduce another food group. During this time, keep a journal of which foods you reintroduced and how you felt throughout the day. Be detailed and really pay attention to any symptoms. This could include feeling fatigued at 2 p.m. after your lunch, getting a bit of a headache around 5 p.m., or having trouble falling asleep. In the beginning you may not be able to describe exactly how you feel, so you can use a numbering system instead. The numbers could go from 1 (poor) to 10 (excellent). Get out a calendar, journal, or spiral notebook and number the days. Add the times of day so you can be very specific about how you react to the foods you eat throughout the day. Don't forget to create a column for comments on how you feel. See page 225 for a sample chart.

You don't have to reintroduce all of these food groups—you could eliminate some of them permanently. If you decide not to reintroduce a particular food group, just skip to the next one.

Day 28: Meat products
Red meat, poultry, pork, eggs, fish (including shellfish)

Day 31: Dairy products
Cheese, milk, yogurt, cottage cheese, sour cream, ice cream

Day 34: Gluten
Wheat, barley, rye, bulgur, durum, farina, graham flour, kamut, semolina, spelt, wheat beer, refined sugary foods and pastries (doughnuts, cookies, cakes)

Day 37: Caffeine
Coffee, tea, soda, chocolate

Day 40: Soy (unfermented)
Tofu, soy protein, soymilk, soybean oil, soy lecithin, soy flour, soy cheese, soy yogurt, soy ice cream, soy "meat," edamame, TVP (texturized vegetable protein)

Day 43: Completion and reflection
Once you have completed the reintroduction phase, look back at your journal to see what foods may have caused adverse reactions. If you note any problem foods, I recommend that you eliminate them from your diet.

A note on food intolerances: If you find that you have an intolerance to a certain food or food group, I urge you to look at the quality of that food. Often, the intolerance is to the toxic nature of the food in the form you are eating it rather than the actual biochemical makeup of the food itself. What exactly does that mean?

A good example is wheat. It has become one of the most highly processed foods, no longer in its pure form but instead in a toxic, immune-compromising form. Wheat is almost always refined, stripped of its beneficial nutrients and husk, and ground into flour. Often, it is fortified with synthetic nutrients that are difficult for the body to use, causing more stress than benefit. Refined wheat products are not sprouted, and sprouting is an important process that eliminates wheat's natural enzyme inhibitors. These inhibitors prevent us from absorbing its nutrients. In addition, a large portion of American-grown wheat is genetically modified, which risks altering the metabolism, reducing fertility, causing inflammation, and adversely affecting kidney and liver function. Finally, a common practice is to use mercury fumigants on wheat or to store it in carbon dioxide containers, therefore exposing consumers to harmful heavy metals and chemicals. It is no wonder that the body is intolerant to wheat when it is laden with toxins and completely stripped of beneficial nutrients.

My recommendation is to completely avoid processed wheat and flour products. Eat organic sprouted wheat products to see if the intolerance is a true allergy or just an immune reaction to the toxic form of wheat you are consuming. You can apply this same concept to other foods such as dairy. Test your tolerance with good dairy like raw, organic, and fermented products such as yogurt, aged cheese, and kefir. Avoid pasteurized, conventional forms like milk, ice cream, and young cheese.

Is Going Back to All the Eliminated Foods Okay?

Say that you passed the food intolerance test with flying colors and don't seem to have an issue eating these foods. Does that make them okay to eat? I bet you have a sneaking suspicion the answer is no.

Sorry to prove you correct, but the foods that you eliminated during the cleanse were eliminated for a reason. They stress the kidneys, and they can be toxic to the body in other ways too. Even if you don't have an intolerance to a food, that does not mean it is a healthy choice. You must consider a few factors when deciding whether a food is healthy or not. There is the actual biochemical makeup of the food, how it is grown or raised (conventional or organic), and how a processed food is made. For example, compare apples sprayed with pesticides, picked too early, then combined with sugar and preservatives with organic apples picked right from the tree; or compare highly heated granola rich in chemical additives with raw, organic granola. I suggest that if you are going to reintroduce the foods that were eliminated, be mindful of what you are purchasing and how often you are eating them.

I will give you a hall pass for a decadent chocolate dessert or a nice glass of wine on special occasions. However, if you are dealing with a kidney disease or condition, most likely you will have to be much stricter about your "cheat" days.

STEP 2: MAKING THE RIGHT FOOD CHOICES

The following is a list of guidelines that will help you navigate a world of cafés, fast-food restaurants, and supermarket aisles filled with enticing products and their emotionally fueled slogans such as "every dinner should feel this good" and "help yourself to happiness."

The Healthy Eating Tenets

1. Eat primarily plant-based foods such as whole grains, raw nuts and seeds, vegetables, fruits, and legumes. Use the Kidney Cleanse Shopping List (page 213) as a guide.

2. Eat local, organic, and seasonal foods. Shop at health food stores and farmer's markets. Remember, the closer to the earth, the healthier the food.

3. Eat as much raw food as possible (fruits, vegetables, nuts, seeds, oils, and seaweeds).

4. If eating animal protein, choose organic and sustainably raised foods (free of antibiotics, hormones, arsenic, chlorine, and pathogens). Look for the following terms on labels:

   EGGS: Free-range, grass-fed, pastured

   DAIRY: Raw, organic

   RED MEAT: Grass-fed, organic

   POULTRY: Grass-fed, free-range, cage-free

   FISH: Wild, not farm-raised. Eat only smaller fish, which have lower levels of mercury

5. Avoid "convenience" foods (microwave meals, canned, packaged, and premade) and food products containing additives, preservatives, and dyes. Avoid the following:

- High-fructose corn syrup, regular corn syrup
- Artificial sweeteners
- MSG (monosodium glutamate)
- Food dyes
- Sodium sulfite, sodium benzoate
- Sodium nitrate, sodium nitrite
- BHA (butylated hydroxyanisole), BHT (butylated hydroxytoluene)
- Sulfur dioxide
- Potassium bromate

6. Eat the right types of fat (coconut, avocado, flax, borage, olive, chia). Avoid highly heated fats (roasted or fried) and the following bad fats:

- Trans fats (hydrogenated or polyunsaturated fat/oil, shortening)
- Vegetable oil
- Canola oil
- Soybean oil
- Margarine
- Butter substitutes

7. Include some of these superfoods in your daily diet:

- Avocado
- Raw nuts and seeds
- Blueberries
- Raw cacao
- Pomegranate
- Kale
- Spinach
- Goji berries
- Coconut oil, coconut butter
- Chia seeds
- Hemp seeds
- Greens powder (chlorella, blue green algae, wheat grass, oat grass)
- Aloe vera
- Bee pollen
- Raw honey
- Maca (a root native to Peru that acts as a powerful adaptogen, increasing energy and helping the body to overcome stress)
- Cacao
- Seaweed
- Camu camu (a berry from the Amazonian rain forest that contains extremely high levels of vitamin C and also supports energy, immune health, and the adrenal glands)
- Flax
- Acai

8. Include some foods rich in probiotics, the healthy bacteria in our gut:

- Sauerkraut
- Kombucha (a fermented, enzyme- and probiotic-rich tea used for digestion and a strong immune system)
- Organic miso
- Organic raw yogurt and kefir
- Kimchi
- Pickled vegetables
- Organic tempeh
- Organic nama shoyu (raw, unpasteurized soy sauce)

9. Eat only nature's candy (dates, figs, raw honey, grade B or #2 maple syrup, molasses, yacon syrup, coconut sugar). Avoid refined sugars (high-fructose corn syrup, white sugar).

10. Avoid foods that are highly heated. High heat damages nutrients, reducing their health benefits and also creating harmful carcinogens (cancer-causing agents). This includes packaged, barbecued, roasted, and fried foods. A few common foods to avoid are roasted nuts, unsprouted conventional breads and crackers, grilled meat and fish, potato chips, and french fries.

11. Avoid foods with the words "lite," "low-fat," "fat-free," "sugar-free," or "no sugar added" on the label. What this really means is that other toxic ingredients were added to replace what was taken out.

Healthy eating practices

Stop eating right before you feel full.

Don't eat because you are bored.

Drink half your weight in ounces of purified water daily.

Get in the habit of reading nutrition labels.

Stay out of the middle of the supermarket (this is where refined foods are).

Don't eat something if you don't know how it was made (for example, Froot Loops, Twinkies, Pop Tarts).

Limit "cheat" days to once a week.

Eat at home because it is almost always healthier than eating out.

Control your portions by eating meals in smaller dishes and by doling out portions with measuring cups and spoons.

STEP 3: MINIMIZING YOUR TOXIC EXPOSURE

Now that you've spent all this time clearing out toxins, how will you keep them from accumulating again? Minimize your toxic exposure so you can limit how often you need to cleanse your kidneys. By changing your lifestyle behaviors, you will be able to reduce your toxic load. The following are the main ways in which most people expose themselves to toxins.

1. Food: Follow the healthy eating tenets and you have this covered.

2. Water: Continue drinking purified, filtered water only. If you are traveling with water, make sure to use either a glass or BPA-free plastic water bottle. Shower in pure water as well. Chlorine filters are a must. This is especially important for reducing heavy metal and chemical exposure.

3. Air: Investing in an air purifier is an excellent way to reduce exposure to pesticides, mold and fungus, pet dander, dust mites, pollen, formaldehyde, VOCs (volatile organic compounds), and indoor chemicals.

4. Limit or eliminate alcohol and caffeinated beverages.

5. Avoid recreational drugs and nicotine.

6. Work to reduce or get off pharmaceutical drugs, especially ones that lead to kidney stress or damage listed in "Nephrotoxic Substances" on page 223.

7. Switch to nontoxic personal care and household cleaning products. You can find these at health food stores and online. This is especially important for reducing heavy metal and chemical exposure.

8. Address any possible heavy metal toxicity by eliminating exposure and undergoing a heavy metal cleanse with a trained practitioner. For common exposures, see the list of heavy metals on page 223.

9. Reduce exposure to electromagnetic pollution from cell phones, TVs, and wireless internet.

10. Exercise: Continue exercising at least four times a week for a minimum of 20 minutes.

STEP 4: DOING SEASONAL AND ANNUAL CLEANSES

The concept of annual or seasonal cleaning is already ingrained in most of us. We have routines for cleaning the house, cleaning our teeth, and checking up on our cars, so why was cleansing the body left out of the loop? The good news is that you just finished cleansing your kidneys, so you recognize its importance, but does that mean you are all done?

Cleansing the kidneys is an ongoing process that should become part of your routine, and once in a lifetime or once every 20 years is just not going to cut it. And cleansed intestines and liver/gallbladder go along with cleansed kidneys. So, exactly what should be cleansed and how often?

That depends on you. Each person has different exposures to toxins, different rates at which toxins are cleared, and different obstacles such as disease that generate toxic accumulation. The following is a guide to help you determine which path is best for you and your health.

You'll know which group you fall into if you answer "yes" to at least four of the categories in the classification descriptions. Please note that these are generalizations and other factors may come into play, but this should set you on the right path.

Group 1: General Good Health — Plant-Based Diet

Classification: No diseases or pre-existing health conditions; plant-based diet (minimal or no meat or dairy consumption); regular exercise; no chemical or heavy metal toxicity; no prescription, OTC, or recreational drug use; minimal exposure to chemicals (pesticides, personal and household products); infrequent (a few times a month) consumption of alcohol, refined sugar, white flour, and processed foods; no cigarette smoking

Health goal: Prevent disease, maintain radiant health

Recommendation
- Major cleanse once a year: Alternate kidney cleanse, liver/gallbladder cleanse, and intestinal cleanse
- Mini cleanse every 6 months: 3-day juice feast with adaptogenic herbs

Group 2: General Good Health — Diet Includes Animal Protein

Classification: Same as Group 1, but diet includes the regular consumption of animal protein (dairy, meat, poultry, fish)

Health goal: Prevent disease, maintain radiant health

Recommendation
- Intestinal cleanse and kidney cleanse every year
- Liver/gallbladder cleanse every other year
- Mini cleanse every 6 months: 3-day juice feast with adaptogenic herbs

Group 3: Compromised Health — High Toxic Load

Classification: No diagnosed disease but dealing with symptoms (such as headaches, insomnia, digestive imbalance, psoriasis, chronic fatigue); intermittent exercise; OTC use; no pharmaceutical or recreational drug use; medium exposure to chemicals (pesticides, personal and household products, industrial); more frequent (a few times a week) consumption of alcohol, refined sugar, white flour, and processed foods; consumption of animal protein; cigarette smoking

Health goal: Clear existing symptoms, offset toxic exposure

Recommendation
- Intestinal cleanse and kidney cleanse every year
- Liver/gallbladder cleanse every other year
- Mini cleanse every 3 months: 3-day juice feast with adaptogenic herbs

Group 4: Compromised Health — Very High Toxic Load

Important note: If you are dealing with a disease or a pre-existing condition, you must consult your doctor before undergoing any cleanse, diet change, or fast.

Classification: Diagnosed disease or pre-existing condition; infrequent exercise; OTC and pharmaceutical or recreational drug use; regular exposure to chemicals (pesticides, personal and household products, industrial); daily consumption of alcohol, refined sugar, white flour, and processed foods; consumption of animal protein; cigarette smoking

Health goal: Manage disease/condition, decrease toxic load

Recommendation

- Major cleanse every 6 months: Alternate kidney cleanse, intestinal cleanse, and liver/gallbladder cleanse
- Mini cleanse every week: 1-day juice feast with adaptogenic herbs

Liver/Gallbladder and Intestinal Cleansing

There are a couple of ways to approach effective and safe liver/gallbladder and intestinal cleansing, both of which start with education. I urge you to be discerning in choosing a program because many programs can be harmful, especially if you are dealing with a disease or condition. The best plan is to find a local alternative practitioner to customize a program for you. If that is not an option, I suggest looking into the following companies and books. Remember, always consult your doctor prior to undertaking a cleanse.

Books

The Liver and Gallbladder Miracle Cleanse: An All-Nature, At-Home Flush to Purify and Rejuvenate Your Body by Andreas Moritz

Complete Colon Cleanse: The At-Home Detox Program to Restore Good Health, Boost Vitality, and Ensure Longevity by Dr. Edward F. Group

Supplement Companies

Pure Encapsulations

Premier Research Labs

Recommendations for Ongoing Cleansing

If you follow the recommended cleansing schedule, you might move yourself into another group and reduce the frequency of major and mini cleansing practices.

No matter which group you fall into, the following are excellent ways to further help clear toxins like heavy metals from your body, particularly a daily detox of the liver/gallbladder and blood.

Daily Practices

- Consume a green drink (smoothie or juice) rich in one of the following ingredients: dandelion, kale, spinach, collard greens, arugula, cabbage, wheatgrass, parsley, cilantro, mustard greens, chard, nettles, cucumber. You can also use a greens powder.

- Include cleansing superfoods in your diet: cilantro, parsley, ginger, spirulina, chlorella, garlic, beets, lemon, turmeric, cayenne, and wheatgrass. Note: Parsley, cilantro, and chlorella are natural heavy metal chelators (they help detoxify heavy metals).

- Manage your stress through such practices as yoga, tai chi, and meditation.

- Tongue scraping: An Ayurvedic tradition, tongue scraping is a method used to detoxify the mouth, used to reduce your overall level of toxicity while maintaining a healthy immune system. Purchase at your local health food store and use once daily after brushing your teeth.

- Grounding: This is the practice of standing barefoot on natural soil such as grass, dirt, sand, or a grounding device in order to rebalance the positive-negative charge in the body. Take 5 to 10 minutes daily for this practice.

- Check the pH of your first morning urine, and modify your diet or supplement program to remain alkaline.

- Use supplements (antioxidants, natural detoxifiers, minerals, and digestive support) to make sure your body's detoxification system works well. See my recommendations in "Resources" on page 207.

- Get plenty of sunshine. Vitamin D level is essential to a healthy immune system and the clearance of toxic substances. Aim for 30 minutes daily without sunscreen (maybe longer if you have dark skin). If you are unable to get that amount of sun, then supplementation with vitamin D3 may be necessary. Note: Vitamin D toxicity can lead to kidney damage. If your kidney function is compromised, consult your doctor before taking a supplement.

Weekly Practices

- Infrared or dry-heat sauna
- Castor oil packs (page 106)
- Enema (page 87)
- Dry brushing (page 108)

STEP 5: STAYING MOTIVATED!

If you ask me, this has to be the hardest part of the entire process. It is one thing to commit yourself to a month-long cleanse, but quite another to continue on the right health track day in and day out. Obviously, it is up to you to figure out what works best for you, but I believe the most foolproof practices are as follows:

Join or Create a Health Community

There is nothing better than having someone to share your health journey with, someone standing on the sidelines cheering you on or giving you a much-needed kick in the butt when you don't think you can do it anymore. It doesn't matter whether you call that person your health coach, your health sponsor, your partner in crime, or your insurance policy for lifelong health success.

I know many of you live in areas where eating kale and drinking green juice is either some sort of hippie practice or an anorexic ploy, but there has to be someone for you to share this experience with. Whether you have to search online for "local meet-up groups" or create your own group at a church or synagogue, or the local Y or community center, having the support of others is critical to your ongoing success.

Get together with a group, even if that group is you plus one. You can have weekly or monthly meetings where you share health recipes, drink homemade, fresh-pressed green juice, and talk about your favorite yoga moves and how weird everyone thinks you are. And if you are lucky enough to live in a health hub (such as the Bay Area, Los Angeles, New York City, Austin, or Portland, Oregon), then you have no excuses. Get yourself out there and get involved, because the road is so much more enjoyable and you can cover more ground when you have someone to walk with.

Get Educated — the More You Know, the More Motivated You Are

My belief is that the more you can learn about why you are doing something, the more motivated you are to follow through and reach your goal. In this case, that involves learning about nutrition, the world around you, and how you relate to it. Before you see this as yet another task on your evergrowing list of things to do, I urge you to give it a chance. Learning about health is actually interesting, engaging, and even exciting because it has to do with the one thing we all love learning about—ourselves.

Your reason for taking control of your health may be different from another person's. It may be because you don't want to see animals harmed, you care about the conservation of our planet, you want to make sure to live long enough to see your children marry, or you just want to feel good enough to tear it up on the ski slopes on your next vacation. Whatever your reason, your engagement and a vested interest are key, and knowledge is the path to get you there. Find a way to make that connection and to share it with your new health support club. It might consist of showing a health documentary or learning how to churn butter. Just find something that motivates you!

CHAPTER NINE

SPECIAL PROGRAMS

ADJUSTING THE CLEANSE FOR KIDNEY CONDITIONS

Some of you who have picked up this book are currently dealing with or have dealt with kidney disease or dysfunction, or have a history of kidney disease in your family. Naturally, you are looking for a way to turn your health around or prevent any further problems.

According to the Centers for Disease Control and Prevention, kidney disease is the eighth leading cause of death in America, affecting 1 in 10 adults. And 1 in 11 people suffer from kidney stones. The problem with kidney disease and related conditions is that they are quite complicated. For example, what may improve kidney disease may be harmful to people with a history of kidney stones. Depending on the disease or condition you are tackling, some aspects of this cleanse may not be in your best interest.

I cannot say strongly enough how important it is for you to consult your doctor before starting this cleanse, changing your diet, or taking supplements. The kidneys are extremely responsive to herbs, supplements, and diet, and any changes must be managed by your doctor.

With the caveat that you must talk to your doctor, here's a quick review of the various states of kidney dysfunction, their risk factors, and how you can alter the kidney cleanse, supplementation, and diet to tailor the program to your needs. Remember, these are mere guidelines and are not intended as a cure for any disease or condition.

KIDNEY STONES (RENAL CALCULUS, NEPHROLITHIASIS)

A kidney stone is a crystalized aggregation or hard mass that ranges in size and shape. A stone develops because of factors that include mineral buildup and infection. Specific therapies must be used to target stones based on cause. Still, the number-one recommendation for all types of stones is increasing water intake and in turn urine volume. Residual mineral fragments, or "seeds," are often left in the kidney and, if not flushed out by urine, can grow into a kidney stone. Increasing your hydration so that you produce 2 to 3 liters of urine a day will have a profound influence on the prevention of kidney stones.

The following is an outline that will help you to understand the risk factors of developing kidney stones, how you can reduce your risk, and how to make the necessary alterations to the kidney cleanse diet to address a current history of stones.

1. CALCIUM STONES (OXALATE, PHOSPHATE, APATITE, BRUSHITE)

Prevalence: Most common, 60 to 80% of kidney stones

Specific risk factors leading to development:
- Calcium intake from supplementation
- Low intake of calcium from dietary sources
- Exposure to fluoride
- Low (acidic) pH
- Regular consumption of apple or grapefruit juice
- Diseases: distal renal tubular acidosis, Dent disease, hyperparathyroidism, primary hyperoxaluria, medullary sponge kidney, Crohn's disease, ileal bypass surgery

Specific antagonists to development (tools for prevention):
- Supplementation with potassium citrate
- Low-sodium diet (less than 2,300 mg/day)
- Low-oxalate diet (less than 50 mg/day)
- Limited vitamin C supplementation (may increase oxalates)
- Oxalobacter formigenes (probiotic)

Kidney cleanse strategy:
- Substitute pears for apples in juice recipes.
- Avoid high-oxalate foods (see the food list on page 202).
- Drink Kidney Cleanse Juice #1 daily. It contains potato, an excellent source of citrate.

Supplementation:
- Include an antioxidant supplement, such as alpha lipoic acid, in your regimen. Stones begin to form after toxic agents cause free radical damage to the kidney cells, and antioxidants battle free radicals.
- It may also be beneficial to supplement with a probiotic containing the beneficial bacteria Oxalobacter formigenes.
- Vitamin B6 (more than 40 mg/day) and magnesium (400 mg/day) are recommended for the prevention of oxalate stone production.
- Omega-3 fatty acids are thought to reduce the excretion of calcium in the kidneys, thus reducing stone development.
- If you are on diuretics or use herbs that have a diuretic effect, consider supplementing with potassium magnesium citrate.

2. STRUVITE (TRIPLE PHOSPHATE) STONES

Prevalence: 10 to 15% of kidney stones

Specific risk factors leading to development:
- Urinary tract infection from urea-splitting bacteria (Proteus, Klebsiella, Serratia, Mycoplasma), which cause alkaline urine.

Specific antagonists to development (tools for prevention):
- Lowered urine pH (5.5–5.6)

Kidney cleanse strategy:
- Drink cranberry juice daily to acidify your urine.
- Supplementation with hyssop has shown some promise in addressing urinary tract infections.

3. URIC ACID OR URATE STONES

Prevalence: 5 to 10% of kidney stones

Specific risk factors leading to development:
- Low (acidic) pH—important risk factor
- Hyperuricaemia, hyperuricosuria, or gout—doubles the risk
- High uric acid (metabolizes from purines in wine, red meat, and similar)
- Low urine volume
- Infection with urease-producing bacteria (Staphylococcus, Klebsiella, Ureaplasma urealyticum, Pseudomonas, or Providencia)
- High excretion of sodium in urine

Specific antagonists to development (tools for prevention):
- Hydration
- Raised urine pH (6.5–7.0)
- Low purine diet
- Supplementation with potassium citrate

Kidney cleanse strategy:
- Avoid high-purine foods (page 203).
- Drink kidney cleanse juice #1 daily. It contains potato, an excellent source of potassium citrate.
- Eat black and/or tart cherries, either in juices, smoothies, or on their own.
- Supplementation with folic acid and niacin (vitamin B3) has been shown to be beneficial in reducing uric acid buildup. Omega-3 fatty acids are also essential.

4. CYSTINE STONES

Prevalence: 1 to 2% of kidney stones

Specific risk factors leading to development:
- Genetic defect of the nephron-impairing renal absorption of amino acids, specifically cystine

Specific antagonists (tools for prevention):

- Raised urine pH (7.5–8)
- Increased urine volume (hydration)
- Diet low in sodium and animal protein
- Supplementation with potassium citrate

Kidney cleanse strategy:

- Drink Kidney Cleanse Juice #1 daily. It contains potato juice, an excellent source of potassium citrate.
- Increase water consumption until you are passing 3 to 4 liters of urine a day.
- Eat a diet low in methionine-rich and cysteine-rich foods. (See the food lists on page 202.)
- Reduce intake of dietary sodium. (See the list of high-sodium foods on page 201.)

BREAKING THE STONES

The growing prevalence of kidney stones (1 in 11 people in the United States suffers from them) could be considered a mini-epidemic. While the kidney cleanse is a tool to prevent kidney stones from developing, what can you do if you currently have a kidney stone? The process of breaking down kidney stones can stress the kidneys and can even be dangerous if not done properly, so please use the following information under your doctor's guidance.

Chanca Piedra (*Phyllanthus niruri*)

Chanca piedra is a tropical plant whose other common name is "stone breaker." It is an herb used by indigenous people in the Amazon River region to eliminate gallstones and kidney stones.

The plant facilitates the expulsion of kidney stones by acting as a potent antispasmodic, allowing the smooth muscle tissues of the ureter and bladder walls to relax. Once the tissues relax, the stones can pass through the urinary canal with ease. Chanca piedra is even thought to prevent stones from forming. A 1999 lab study at a Brazilian medical school indicated the plant's ability to inhibit the production of calcium oxalate crystals.

Chanca piedra has been shown to have no side effects other than possible cramping from the expulsion of the stones. Please use this herb only under your doctor's guidance because the correct dosage is key to preventing any damage. Also, the herb has been reported to have interactions with some medications and shouldn't be taken with them.

Both research and clinical evidence back the use of chanca piedra for kidney stones. I have worked with many practitioners who have had success with chanca piedra, but the most notable clinical evidence is from researcher Nicole Maxwell. She reported that Dr. Wolfram Wiemann of Nuremburg, Germany, treated more than a hundred kidney stone patients with chanca piedra obtained in Peru and found it to be 94% successful in eliminating stones within a week or two.

In addition to chanca piedra's use in breaking up kidney stones and gallstones, its other applications include the following:

- Cellular and liver protection
- Lower high blood pressure (hypertension)
- Lower cholesterol levels
- Analgesic (pain relief)
- Antiviral

An interesting aspect of chanca piedra is its use for combating high cholesterol and high blood pressure because both are risk factors for kidney disease. Chanca piedra may prove to be integral in an integrated approach for people at high risk for both kidney disease and kidney stones.

Recommendation: Royal Break-Stone by Whole World Botanicals

ACUTE RENAL FAILURE (ARF)

This is a form of rapid kidney failure in which the kidneys stop functioning properly due to sudden illness, medication, or a medical condition. There are three types of ARF: prerenal, intrarenal, and postrenal. When ARF is treated right away, more than 80% of that kidney function will be recovered, making it vital to support the kidneys during this acute time.

1. PRERENAL ARF

This is due to decreased blood flow to the kidneys where there was no inherent problem with the kidneys beforehand. Prerenal ARF can usually be reversed as long as inadequate blood flow does not continue for more than a few hours, in which case intrarenal ARF will occur.

Risk factors:

- Heart failure with reduced cardiac output and low blood pressure
- Major surgery
- Severe burns with fluid loss
- Massive bleeding (hemorrhage)
- Heart attack
- Blood clots

2. INTRARENAL OR INTRINSIC ARF

This is kidney tissue damage that leads to impaired glomerular filtration and tubular function.

Risk factors:

- Disease (tubular, glomerular, vascular, interstitial)
- Damage to filtering units from glomerulonephritis, toxic chemicals, medications, or infection

Forms of intrarenal ARF:

- Acute nephritic syndrome (glomerulonephritis); 95% of cases occur after an infection (staphylococcal and gram-negative bacteria) elsewhere in the body
- Acute tubular necrosis (due to renal ischemia, prolonged or unresolved prerenal ARF); can be caused by poisons, heavy metals, chemical toxins such as pesticides, or medications
- Interstitial nephritis; caused by bacterial infections from the bladder (E. coli), or a reaction to a medication or other diseases or toxins that damage the kidneys

3. POSTRENAL ARF

This is due to a blockage of urine flow after it has left the kidneys.

Risk factors:

- Kidney stones
- Obstruction from tumor (bladder, cervix, prostate)
- Retroperitoneal fibrosis
- Urethral obstruction secondary to an enlarged prostate

CHRONIC KIDNEY DISEASE

Chronic kidney disease (CKD), also called chronic renal failure, is due to the loss of a large number of nephrons, the basic functioning units of the kidney, over time. This results in a decreased glomerular filtration rate (GFR), or flow rate of filtered fluid through the kidneys, and the ability for the glomeruli to filter and excrete waste products.

Chronic kidney disease is divided into stages based on GFR. Normal is roughly greater than 90, while less than 60 is considered CKD, with or without the known presence of kidney damage. Stage 1 is the mildest, causing the least symptoms and having the highest chance of recovery, while stage 5 is the most severe, with little chance of recovery and requiring dialysis. Clinical symptoms occur when less than 30% of nephrons function. These nephron units must take on the work of the missing 70%.

Risk factors:

- Diabetic nephropathy
- High blood pressure (hypertension) and hardening of the arteries (atherosclerosis)
- Chronic kidney inflammation (glomerulonephritis and pyelonephritis)
- Long-term exposure to metals

KIDNEY CLEANSE STRATEGY

It is vital that you discuss the kidney cleanse with your doctor before you embark on it. The cleanse can be valuable to you and your condition, but it must be monitored. In addition to following the general guidelines of the kidney cleanse, you must increase your antioxidant levels.

Antioxidants are substances that prevent damage to the body's cells, tissues, and organs from free radicals, which result from oxidation. Get it, "anti" and "oxidant"—prevention against oxidation? Antioxidants act as police, putting away the bad guys before they do any harm, and they also act as builders and contractors, fixing any damage. Unfortunately, kidney dysfunction leaves the body deficient in many of naturally occurring antioxidants, leading to cell and tissue damage. To prevent this damage, you must increase your antioxidant levels through the kidney cleanse food plan and supplementation. Here are lists of antioxidants, most of them available in foods, that have been shown to help the kidneys.

For end-stage renal disease (ESRD):
- Vitamin C: camu camu, citrus, papaya, pineapple, brussels sprouts, broccoli, kale, cantaloupe, bell peppers, kiwi
- Selenium: Brazil nuts, wild salmon, barley, cod, lamb, sardines, walnuts, legumes
- Vitamin E: sunflower seeds, almonds, spinach, chard, mustard greens, collard greens, asparagus, bell peppers, rice bran
- Glutathione: nutritional yeast, rice bran, turmeric, avocados, tomatoes, spinach, garlic, asparagus, broccoli, walnuts
- B vitamins: nutritional yeast, fruits, vegetables

For all forms of kidney dysfunction, the following are recommended:
- Ginseng saponin
- Curcumin (turmeric)
- Wild blueberries
- Coenzyme Q10
- Quercetin: capers, tarragon, spring onion, red onion, Serrano pepper, dill, cranberries, buckwheat
- Alpha lipoic acid (ALA)
- Ginkgo biloba
- Omega-3 fatty acids (DHA/EPA blend): wild salmon, sardines, grass-fed beef, walnuts, hemp seeds, chia seeds, flaxseeds

I am sure you are wondering if it is necessary to take all of the antioxidants on this second list, for all forms of kidney dysfunction, every day. Daily consumption is ideal. That may mean taking some as supplements and some in the form of food. Turmeric, blueberries, omega-3 fatty acids, and quercetin are all available in whole foods. This leaves coenzyme Q10, ALA, *Ginkgo biloba*, and ginseng to be taken as supplements. The nice thing is that you may even be able to take complex supplements containing these antioxidants in one or two formulas. For example, Pure Encapsulations makes Revital Age Ultra, which contains coenzyme Q10, ALA, and a wild blueberry concentrate.

If your condition is advanced and severe, ideally take the antioxidants in supplements as well as in food form. Supplements give you higher dosages of the antioxidants than if you ate just a few blueberries or a handful of nuts daily. And to make sure you get enough antioxidants, I recommend that you continue juicing and drinking superfood smoothies daily, because they are an easy way to get your daily fix.

SPECIALIZED SUPPLEMENT THERAPY

Some kidney conditions and those that affect the kidney directly require specialized targeted nutrients. Based on the research done by Sharol Tilgner, N.D., the following is an overview to guide you to the most appropriate formulas for your needs.

Renal anemia
- Deer antler velvet

Uremic syndrome
- Bilberry (*vaccinium myrtillus*)

Dialysis
- Coenzyme Q10
- Carnitine

Dialysis-induced itching
- Capsicum (hot pepper)

Suppressed proteinuria
- Perilla frutescens
- Rosmarinic acid (oil from rosemary, oregano, sage, thyme, or peppermint)

Diabetic nephropathy
- Alpha lipoic acid (ALA)
- Chard leaves
- Carnitine
- Coenzyme Q10
- Vitamin E
- Omega-3 fatty acids

Renal cancer
- Curcumin (turmeric)

Kidney transplant
- Coenzyme Q10
- *Cordyceps sinensis*
- *Ginkgo biloba*
- Omega-3 fatty acids
- Alpha lipoic acid (ALA) during pretreatment
- Quercetin
- Curcumin (turmeric)

IgA nephropathy
- *Cordyceps sinensis*

High blood pressure (hypertension)
- Corn silk
- *Ginkgo biloba*

Hypercholesterolemia due to renal failure
- Allium (garlic)
- Coenzyme Q10

Damage due to toxins (environmental, drugs)
- Coenzyme Q10
- *Cordyceps sinensis*
- Selenium
- Vitamin E
- Vitamin C
- Silymarin (milk thistle)

VITAMIN D DEFICIENCY AND CHRONIC KIDNEY DISEASE

Emerging evidence suggests that the progression of chronic kidney disease and cardiovascular complications may be linked to low vitamin D levels. Vitamin D is essential in maintaining mineral balance, which is impaired in chronic kidney disease. Furthermore, vitamin D has shown to be integral to the prevention of many conditions such as hyperparathyroidism (abnormally high level of parathyroid hormone), high blood pressure, immune disorders, kidney and cardiovascular damage, and bone loss. It is also instrumental in calcium absorption, making adequate levels of vitamin D vital for the prevention of osteopenia and osteoporsis. The current recommendation for people with chronic kidney disease is to supplement with vitamin D, specifically vitamin D3.

When choosing a form of vitamin D3, always choose a live-source form that has not been extracted with hexane. For optimal use by the body, choose a liquid product in which the vitamin D is suspended in organic olive oil.

Recommendation: D3 Gold by Quantum Nutrition Labs

THE PARATHYROID CONNECTION

If I haven't made it crystal clear yet, one of the main functions of the kidneys is to regulate mineral balance, including that of calcium. It's important to address the other players in mineral balance—the parathyroid glands.

The major function of the four parathyroid glands is to regulate the amount of calcium in the body. The glands release parathyroid hormone (PTH), which increases the amount of blood calcium by influencing its breakdown from bone and increasing the absorption of calcium in the gastrointestinal tract. PTH also increases reabsorption of calcium and magnesium and the excretion of phosphorus and bicarbonate in the kidneys. Because the parathyroid plays a significant role in kidney function, it should be addressed as an adjunct to the kidney cleanse. I want to cover all of the bases for you, especially if your goal is to optimize kidney function.

PARATHYROID DYSFUNCTION: KIDNEY STONES AND KIDNEY DISEASE

When the parathyroid is not working properly, the levels of PTH get out of balance, which adversely affects the kidneys. In hyperparathyroidism, too much PTH is secreted, resulting in high amounts of calcium in the blood. Since the kidneys filter calcium, high levels can stress them and calcium may collect in the tubules, leading to kidney stones. In some extreme cases, the kidneys can become calcified and even take on the characteristics of bone.

Signs and symptoms of hyperparathyroidism:

- Depression
- Fatigue
- Muscle fatigue
- Mental confusion, lack of concentration
- Abnormal thirst
- Loss of appetite, nausea
- Constipation
- Stomach pain
- Illness with no apparent cause
- Kidney stones
- High blood pressure
- Osteopenia or osteoporosis
- Acid reflux
- Heart palpitations

In hypoparathyroidism, too little PTH is secreted, resulting in low levels of calcium and high levels of phosphorus in the blood. This condition is managed with calcium supplements, which must be carefully monitored to prevent kidney damage. The high levels of phosphorus can be especially damaging for anyone dealing with kidney disease.

Warning signs of hypoparathyroidism:

- Tingling in the hands or feet or around the mouth (paresthesia)
- Abnormal muscle movements (jerking, twitching)
- Muscle cramping or spasms
- Fatigue, irritability, anxiety, depression
- Bone pain
- Insomnia

Radiation exposure and parathyroid health

Many factors can lead to parathyroid dysfunction, but one that I want to be sure to mention is radiation exposure. Exposure has become far-reaching and ranges from routine X-rays and airport security screenings to environmental contamination from nuclear testing and disasters. The effects of radiation on the body can cause an increased risk of leukemia and thyroid disease.

One of the lesser known effects is radiation's tie to parathyroid damage. The parathyroid is radiation sensitive. Studies have shown that radiation increases the level of PTH, which can lead to kidney stones. I urge you to ask your doctor about hyperparathyroidism if you are dealing with chronic kidney stones and have been exposed to radiation. My other recommendation is to minimize your exposure to radiation if you can. If you can't, be sure to get nutrients that offset the impact of radiation on your body.

Note: The thyroid gland is also radiation sensitive, so when you protect your parathyroid from radiation, you're also protecting your thyroid.

Common sources of radiation exposure:

- X-rays and CT scans
- Airplane travel
- Tobacco products
- Natural gas in the home
- Building materials (brick, cement blocks, granite counter tops, and glazed tiles
- Tap and well water
- Radioactive waste from nuclear plants and military use
- Areas of nuclear disaster

Protective nutrients for radiation exposure:

- Vitamins A, C, and E
- Selenium
- Melatonin
- Polyphenols in green tea
- Iodine
- Potassium iodide
- Zeolite
- Bentonite clay (smectite form)

CHAPTER TEN

RECIPES

In this chapter you'll find a treasure trove of recipes to help you stay satisfied during your kidney cleanse and keep you stocked with fresh ideas for after you transition off the cleanse and into a new, healthier life. The first recipes are specifically designed to help you during your cleansing juice feast, and you'll be sure to find something here that tickles your taste buds as it rids your body of toxins. Don't be afraid to try a new flavor—it just might become your favorite!

JUICE FEAST RECIPES

All juice feast recipes make 1 (16-ounce) serving.

KIDNEY CLEANSE JUICE #1

1 medium russet potato, peeled and chopped (about 2 cups)

2 juicing oranges, peeled

1 bunch cilantro (about 1 cup leaves)

1 medium lemon, peeled

1 garlic clove, peeled

1 medium jalapeño chile pepper, stemmed and seeded

Pass all the ingredients through a juicer.

KIDNEY CLEANSE JUICE #2

2 medium green apples

1 lime, peeled

½ medium field cucumber or 2 Persian cucumbers, peeled

5 celery ribs

½ cup dandelion greens

1 knob ginger (1 x 1 inch), peeled

Pass all the ingredients through a juicer.

KIDNEY CLEANSE JUICE #3

4 celery ribs
1 medium lemon, peeled
2 cups dandelion greens
1 knob ginger (1 x 1 inch), peeled

1 cup parsley leaves
3 cups (15 ounces) chopped watermelon
1 teaspoon apple cider vinegar
⅛ teaspoon sea salt

Pass the celery, lemon, dandelion greens, ginger, parsley, and watermelon through a juicer. Then stir in the apple cider vinegar and salt.

KIDNEY CLEANSE JUICE #4

½ medium pineapple, peeled and chopped (about 2 cups)
2 limes, peeled
1 bunch kale, chopped (about 3 cups)

1 medium lemon, peeled
1 cup parsley leaves
⅛ teaspoon sea salt

Pass the pineapple, limes, kale, lemon, and parsley through a juicer. Stir in the sea salt.

KIDNEY CLEANSE JUICE #5

3 medium lemons, peeled
4 carrots, peeled (about 1 pound)
1 cup peeled and chopped pineapple
½ medium field cucumber, peeled

4 celery ribs
1 knob ginger (1 x 1 inch), peeled
pinch of sea salt

Pass the lemons, carrots, pineapple, cucumber, celery, and ginger through a juicer. Stir in the sea salt.

OTHER JUICES

CUCUMBER MINT JUICE

1 medium field cucumber, peeled and halved
1 bunch mint (about 1 cup leaves)

1 medium lemon, peeled (Meyer lemon is ideal)
1 medium apple (Gala, Pink Lady, or Fuji)

Pass all the ingredients through a juicer.

PEAR JUICE

1 medium pear (any variety)
1 bunch parsley (about 1 cup leaves)
1 medium cucumber, peeled

1 medium lemon, peeled
1 knob ginger (1 x 1 inch), peeled

Pass all the ingredients through a juicer.

TURMERIC TONIC

2 medium carrots, peeled
½ cup cilantro leaves
1 knob ginger (1 x 1 inch), peeled
¼ teaspoon turmeric

10 ounces coconut water
pinch of cayenne
pinch of sea salt

Pass the carrots, cilantro, and ginger through a juicer. Stir in the turmeric, coconut water, cayenne, and sea salt.

WATERMELON LIME JUICE

2–3 cups cubed watermelon
1 bunch parsley (about 1 cup leaves)
1 lime, peeled

1 medium lemon, peeled (Meyer is lemon is ideal)
1 knob ginger (1 x 1 inch), peeled

Pass all the ingredients through a juicer.

CELERY PEAR JUICE

7 celery ribs
1 medium pear (any variety)

½ medium cucumber, peeled
1 (2-inch) knob ginger, peeled

Pass all the ingredients through a juicer.

GREEN APPLE CELERY JUICE

2 medium green apples
7 celery ribs

Pass the apples and celery through a juicer.

CUCUMBER TROPICAL COOLER

1 medium cucumber, peeled
1 cup peeled and chopped pineapple

1 bunch mint
3 ounces coconut water

Juice the cucumber, pineapple, and mint, then stir coconut water into the juice.

SUPERFOOD SMOOTHIES

Choose from the following recipes to make your breakfast daily. If you do not have an ingredient on hand or do not want to eat it, feel free to make a substitution. The following ingredients can easily be interchanged.

USE THIS...	...OR THIS
Banana	Avocado
Greens powder	1 cup dense greens (kale or spinach) or 1 teaspoon blue green algae or chlorella
Coconut butter	Coconut oil
Protein powder (about 1 tablespoon)	½ cup raw nuts (Brazil nuts, almonds, walnuts), preferably soaked
Coconut water	Filtered water
Almond milk	Other vegan milks (hemp, rice, coconut), coconut water, filtered water
Hemp seeds	Chia seeds or flaxseeds
Raw honey	Stevia, grade B or #2 maple syrup, yacon syrup, molasses
Blueberries	Raspberries, strawberries, cranberries
Almond butter, raw	Other raw nut butters (cashew, macadamia, pistachio, pecan, walnut) excluding peanut

Other tips:

If you would like the smoothie to be thicker (and more filling), choose from the following: ice, raw nuts or nut butter, coconut butter, chia seeds, vegan milk, frozen banana, avocado.

If you would like the smoothie to be sweeter, choose from the following: banana, dates, molasses, grade B or #2 maple syrup, yacon syrup, stevia, vanilla extract, raw honey.

If you would like the smoothie to be thinner, add more water or coconut water.

Vegan protein powder: For a sweeter flavor I recommend using vanilla protein powder, which reduces the need for other sweeteners.

To ensure a creamy smoothie: If your blender isn't very powerful, then it's important to chop the vegetables and herbs and to mince the ginger. If you are using a high-speed blender like a Vitamix, then you should be able to add the herbs and vegetables without chopping, mincing, or dicing.

All smoothie recipes make 1 (2-cup) serving

BERRY GREEN SMOOTHIE

1 ½ cups water
1 small cucumber, peeled
½ cup blueberries
½ medium avocado, peeled and pitted
2 celery ribs
1 tablespoon hemp seeds
1 tablespoon greens powder
stevia, to taste

Blend all the ingredients in a high-speed blender until creamy.

ORANGE LASSI SMOOTHIE

1 cup unsweetened almond milk
1 cup ice cubes
1 teaspoon vanilla extract
2 oranges, peeled (any variety)
1 medium lemon, peeled (Meyer lemon is ideal)
1 (2-tablespoon) scoop protein powder
1 teaspoon coconut butter
1 tablespoon tahini
¼ teaspoon turmeric
1 knob (1 x 1 inch) ginger, peeled and sliced
pinch of sea salt
½ medium banana (optional, for extra sweetness)

Blend all the ingredients in a high-speed blender until creamy.

KIDNEY CLEANSING SMOOTHIE

1 ½ cups unsweetened almond milk
1 medium lemon, peeled
1 lime, peeled
½ medium avocado, peeled and pitted
¼ cup chopped dandelion greens
1 knob ginger (1 x 1 inch), peeled
1 medium banana

Blend all the ingredients in a high-speed blender until creamy.

GREEN WATERMELON SMOOTHIE

1 cup water

2 cups cubed watermelon

1 lime, peeled

1 medium lemon, peeled

1 small cucumber, peeled

1 knob ginger (1 x 1 inch), peeled

½ cup mint leaves

1 medium banana

1 tablespoon hemp seeds

1 (2-tablespoon) scoop protein powder

1 cup chopped kale

Blend all the ingredients in a high-speed blender until creamy.

DANDELION SMOOTHIE

1 ½ cups unsweetened almond milk

1 medium lemon, peeled (Meyer lemon is ideal)

1 lime, peeled

½ medium avocado, peeled and pitted

½ cup parsley leaves

¼ cup chopped dandelion greens

1 knob ginger (1 x 1 inch), peeled

1 medium banana

1 teaspoon coconut butter

1 tablespoon hemp seeds

stevia (optional, to sweeten)

Blend all the ingredients in a high-speed blender until creamy.

CUCUMBER AVOCADO SMOOTHIE

1 ½ cups water

2 Persian cucumber or ½ medium field cucumber, peeled

½ medium avocado, peeled and pitted

1 lime, peeled

1 medium lemon, peeled

1 (2-tablespoon) scoop protein powder

1 teaspoon vanilla extract

1 teaspoon chopped fresh parsley

1 tablespoon chia seeds

1 tablespoon hemp seeds

1 teaspoon coconut butter

Blend all the ingredients in a high-speed blender until creamy.

CASHEW BLUEBERRY SMOOTHIE

1 ½ cups water

¼ cup raw cashews

1 medium banana

½ cup blueberries

1 (2-tablespoon) scoop protein powder

1 medium lemon, peeled

1 tablespoon chia seeds

½ teaspoon vanilla extract

pinch of sea salt

Blend all the ingredients in a high-speed blender until creamy.

ALMOND FIG SMOOTHIE

1 ½ cups unsweetened almond milk
3 fresh figs
½ cup blueberries
1 teaspoon coconut butter

1 tablespoon chia seeds
1 (2-tablespoon) scoop protein powder
1 tablespoon greens powder
pinch of ground cinnamon

Blend all the ingredients in a high-speed blender until creamy.

SWEET PEAR SMOOTHIE

1 ½ cups water
1 medium pear (any variety)
1 medium banana
½ medium avocado, peeled and pitted
2 tablespoons hemp seeds

1 (2-tablespoon) scoop protein powder
½ medium lemon, peeled
1 tablespoon fresh aloe vera juice
pinch of sea salt
pinch of ground cinnamon

Blend all the ingredients in a high-speed blender until creamy.

MINTY GREEN SMOOTHIE

1 ½ cups water
1 large or 2 small bananas
½ medium avocado, peeled and pitted
2 tablespoons hemp seeds
½ medium cucumber, peeled
1 (2-tablespoon) scoop protein powder

1 tablespoon greens powder
2 tablespoons mint leaves
1 tablespoon raw honey
pinch of sea salt

Blend all the ingredients in a high-speed blender until creamy.

CRANBERRY CLEANSING SMOOTHIE

1 cup unsweetened almond milk
½ cup 100% pure unsweetened cranberry juice
2 cups chopped kale

1 tablespoon hemp seeds
¼ cup blueberries
¼ cup raspberries
1 medium banana

Blend all the ingredients in a high-speed blender until creamy.

GREEN JUICE SMOOTHIE

1 medium cucumber, peeled

3 celery ribs

1 medium lemon, peeled

½ cup unsweetened almond milk

1 medium banana

1 (2-tablespoon) scoop protein powder

1 tablespoon hemp seeds

1 tablespoon chia seeds

1 teaspoon coconut butter

Juice the cucumber, celery, and lemon. This should yield about 1½ cups juice. Stir together with the almond milk. In a high-speed blender, combine the juice and milk mixture with the remaining ingredients and blend until creamy.

SWEET GREEN CITRUS SMOOTHIE

1½ cups water

1 large banana

1 large or 2 small lemons, peeled (Meyer lemon is ideal)

1 cup baby spinach leaves

1 teaspoon coconut butter

1 tablespoon chia seeds

1 tablespoon hemp seeds

Blend all the ingredients in a high-speed blender until creamy.

BLACK CHERRY SMOOTHIE

1½ cups unsweetened almond milk

1 medium banana

1 cup pitted black cherries

2 cups chopped spinach or kale leaves

1 tablespoon chia seeds

1 (2-tablespoon) scoop protein powder

pinch of ground cinnamon

1 tablespoon raw honey (optional, for extra sweetness)

Blend all the ingredients in a high-speed blender until creamy.

MINT MOJITO PROTEIN SMOOTHIE

1½ cups coconut water

2 tablespoons hemp seeds

2 cups chopped kale

1–2 limes, peeled (sweet limes are ideal)

½ medium avocado, peeled and pitted

1 (2-tablespoon) scoop vanilla protein powder

1 medium banana

¼ cup mint leaves

pinch of sea salt

Blend all the ingredients in a high-speed blender until creamy.

KEY LIME PIE SMOOTHIE

1 ½ cups unsweetened almond milk

1 medium banana

½ medium avocado, peeled and pitted

2 limes, peeled (sweet limes are ideal)

2 bunches (2 cups) spinach

½ teaspoon vanilla extract

1 (2-tablespoon) scoop vanilla protein powder

Blend all the ingredients in a high-speed blender until creamy.

PARSLEY GREEN SMOOTHIE

1 ½ cups water

½ cup chopped fresh parsley

1 medium lemon, peeled (Meyer lemon is ideal)

1 tablespoon minced fresh ginger

1 medium banana

3 cups kale, chopped

1 (2-tablespoon) scoop vanilla protein powder

1 teaspoon coconut butter

1 teaspoon vanilla extract

1 tablespoon hemp seeds

1 teaspoon raw honey (optional, for extra sweetness)

Blend all the ingredients in a high-speed blender until creamy.

SOUPS AND SALADS

CABBAGE AND LEEK SOUP

Serves 2

1 cup minced fresh dill

½ cup plus 1 tablespoon sun-dried tomato–infused olive oil (or extra virgin olive oil)

3 tablespoons extra virgin olive oil, divided

3 medium leeks, trimmed and thinly sliced

3 medium Yukon Gold potatoes (about 18 ounces), thinly sliced

5 garlic cloves, thinly sliced

2 celery ribs, chopped

½ medium head red cabbage, thinly sliced

1 quart (4 cups) organic vegetable broth (made without canola oil)

2–3 teaspoons sea salt

nutritional yeast, to taste

Combine the dill and sun-dried tomato–infused olive oil in a blender or food processor. Blend until smooth.

In a large soup pot over medium heat, warm 2 tablespoons of the olive oil and 5 tablespoons of the dill-infused oil. Add the leeks and cover. Make sure the oil is not bubbling; if it is, turn the heat down. After 5 to 8 minutes, or when the leeks begin to soften, add the potatoes, garlic, celery, and cabbage. Cook for 15 minutes, covered, stirring regularly to make sure the vegetables are not burning. You may add the remaining tablespoon olive oil if the pan dries out. After 15 minutes, when the potatoes begin to soften, stir in the vegetable broth. Make sure the broth is simmering, and then cover. Let cook for another 5 minutes.

At this point the vegetables should be fully cooked; if not, cook for a little longer, then add 2 to 3 teaspoons salt, or to taste. Add the salt at the end. This helps keep the nutrient value high. Serve warm and with the remaining dill-infused oil to taste. Sprinkle with nutritional yeast.

CREAMY BROCCOLI SOUP

Serves 3–4

1–2 tablespoons coconut oil
1 medium sweet onion, chopped
4 garlic cloves, minced
1 cup chopped celery
1½ cups peeled, chopped carrots
1 quart (4 cups) vegetable broth (made without canola oil)
1 cup water

6 cups chopped broccoli
2 tablespoons minced fresh oregano
2 tablespoons Dijon mustard
2 teaspoons sea salt
1 avocado, cut into chunks
3–4 tablespoons chopped fresh chives
black pepper, to taste

In a large soup pot, heat the oil over medium-low heat. Add the onion, garlic, celery, and carrots. Sauté for 5 to 10 minutes, until the vegetables are slightly soft. Add the vegetable broth, water, broccoli, and oregano, and bring to a boil. Reduce the heat, cover, and simmer for about 15 minutes, until the vegetables are tender. Remove from the heat and let cool slightly, about 2 minutes.

Puree the soup in a high-powered blender. Blend in the mustard. You might have to blend the soup in batches if the whole mixture doesn't fit in the blender. Once the soup is thoroughly blended, transfer it back to the soup pot. Stir in salt. To serve, ladle the soup into bowls and top with avocado and chives. Season with black pepper to taste.

ASPARAGUS PUREE WITH ROASTED POTATOES

Serves 2

ROASTED POTATOES	ASPARAGUS PUREE
1 cup sliced fingerling or red potatoes, ¼ inch thick	30 asparagus spears
2 tablespoons extra virgin olive oil	1 tablespoon coconut oil
1 tablespoon fresh minced rosemary	5 garlic cloves, minced
½ teaspoon sea salt	3 tablespoons diced onion
3–4 garlic cloves, minced	3 tablespoons unsweetened almond milk, or more as needed
	sea salt and black pepper to taste

Make the Roasted Potatoes: Preheat the oven to 425°F. Add the potatoes to a roasting pan or baking sheet, and toss with the olive oil, rosemary, sea salt, and garlic so the bottom of the pan and the potatoes are lightly coated. Add more olive oil 1 teaspoon at a time if you feel that the vegetables aren't coated enough, but not too much; you don't want them swimming in olive oil. Bake for 15 to 20 minutes, until the potatoes are tender.

Make the Asparagus Puree: Fill the bottom half of a steamer with water and bring to a boil. Prepare an ice bath by filling a bowl with ice water. Trim the ends off the asparagus spears and place the spears in the top half of the steamer pan. Steam for 5 to 10 minutes, depending on the thickness of the asparagus, or until the asparagus is tender. Then plunge into the ice bath to retain the color. Once the asparagus is cool to the touch, cut the spears into pieces and set aside to cool completely.

Warm the coconut oil in a sauté pan or skillet over medium heat, then add the garlic and onion. Cook, stirring, for about 5 minutes, or until iridescent. Then combine the cooked asparagus, sautéed garlic and onion, and almond milk in a blender or food processor. Blend until creamy. If too thick, slowly add more almond milk to thin. You can use olive oil instead to thin. Season with sea salt and black pepper. Set aside and keep warm.

Serve the asparagus puree in bowls and top with roasted potatoes. Add more sea salt or black pepper if needed.

CREAM OF DANDELION SOUP

Serves 2

6 cups chopped dandelion greens

1 tablespoon extra virgin olive oil

2 garlic cloves, minced

½ medium onion, chopped

2 medium leeks, washed, trimmed and sliced

1 large carrot, peeled and sliced

1 quart (4 cups) vegetable broth

2 ½ cups unsweetened almond milk

1 tablespoon Dijon mustard

sea salt and black pepper, to taste

Bring a large pot of water to a boil and prepare an ice bath by filling a bowl with ice water. When the water boils, briefly plunge the dandelion greens into the boiling water just until they turn bright green, then quickly transfer them to the ice bath to stop the cooking process. Allow to cool.

Heat the oil in a large pot over medium heat and add the garlic and onions. Cook the garlic and onions until they become translucent, 3 to 5 minutes. Then add the dandelion greens along with the leeks and carrots, and cook, stirring, for 15 minutes, until the vegetables soften. Add the vegetable broth and allow to simmer for 15 minutes. Then reduce the heat to low and add the milk. Cook until slightly thick, about 10 minutes.

Transfer the soup to a blender or food processor, and puree until smooth. You might have to blend the soup in batches if the whole mixture doesn't fit in the blender or food processor. Once the soup is thoroughly blended, transfer it back to the soup pot. Add the mustard and season with salt and pepper.

BBQ RANCH SHIITAKE SALAD

Serves 1

"RANCH" DRESSING

½ cup cashews
¼ cup apple cider vinegar
1 garlic clove, minced
¼ teaspoon sea salt
1 tablespoon minced dill
1 tablespoon minced cilantro
¼ cup extra virgin olive oil
2 tablespoons water (optional)

"BBQ" SAUCE

½ cup sun-dried tomatoes
3 tablespoons apple cider vinegar
1 tablespoon miso paste
1 garlic clove, minced
1 tablespoon fresh lemon juice
1 tablespoon molasses or raw honey
¼ teaspoon sea salt
3 tablespoons extra virgin olive oil

SALAD

2 cups romaine or butter lettuce
½ cup Japanese cucumber, diced
½ cup halved cherry tomatoes
6 shiitake mushrooms, sliced
½ medium avocado, peeled, pitted, and diced
½ cup canned black beans, drained and rinsed

Make the "Ranch" Dressing: Combine all the ingredients except the olive oil and water in a blender. Blend on high until creamy. Then slowly add the olive oil and also the water, if needed for consistency, while running the blender on low.

Make the "BBQ" Sauce: Combine all the ingredients except the olive oil in a blender. Blend on high until creamy, then slowly add the olive oil with the blender running on low speed.

Make the Salad: Combine all the salad ingredients in a large bowl, then add the "ranch" dressing and "BBQ" sauce to taste. You will have dressing and sauce left over. Store in an airtight glass container in the refrigerator for one week.

MEXICAN BEAN SALAD

Serves 2

SALAD

2 cups peeled, diced jicama (12 ounces)

1 large avocado, peeled, pitted, and diced

1 (15-ounce) can black beans, drained and rinsed

kernels from 1 ear raw corn

½ cup minced cilantro

1 pint (2 cups) cherry tomatoes, sliced

1 jalapeño chile pepper, seeded and minced

DRESSING

3 tablespoons rice wine vinegar

3 tablespoons extra virgin olive oil

1 tablespoon fresh lime juice

¼ teaspoon sea salt

¼ teaspoon raw honey

¼ teaspoon ground cumin

Toss all the salad ingredients together in a large bowl. In a small bowl, whisk together all the dressing ingredients until thoroughly mixed. Toss the salad with the dressing and serve.

THREE BEAN QUINOA SALAD

Serves 3

SALAD

2 cups raw green beans

1 (15-ounce) can garbanzo beans, drained and rinsed

1 (15-ounce) can kidney beans, drained and rinsed

1 cup chopped green onion

1 cup diced cucumber

½ cup chopped fresh parsley

1 red bell pepper, chopped

1 cup cooked quinoa

DRESSING

6 tablespoons apple cider vinegar

½ cup extra virgin olive oil

2 tablespoons raw honey

4 garlic cloves, roasted

2 teaspoons garlic powder

¼ teaspoon sea salt

Toss all the salad ingredients except the quinoa together in a large bowl. Combine all the dressing ingredients in a blender and puree until smooth, or whisk thoroughly in a medium bowl. Add the quinoa to the bean salad, then toss with the dressing and serve.

SWEET CELERY SALAD

Serves 2 (side dish)

SALAD

- 8 celery ribs, chopped
- 1 cup raw walnuts, soaked for 3 hours
- 4 dates or dried figs, chopped
- 7 red radishes, sliced
- 1 tablespoon chopped fresh parsley
- ½ cup canned white beans, drained and rinsed

DRESSING

- 2 tablespoons rice wine vinegar
- ½ teaspoon raw honey
- ¼ teaspoon sea salt
- ½ teaspoon Dijon mustard
- ½ teaspoon tahini
- 1 tablespoon extra virgin olive oil

Toss all the salad ingredients together in a large bowl. Combine all the dressing ingredients except the oil in a blender. Puree, then slowly add the oil with the blender running on low speed. Toss the salad with the dressing and serve.

BLACK SESAME CUCUMBER SALAD

Serves 2 (side dish)

SAUCE

- 1 tablespoon minced fresh dill
- 1 tablespoon minced fresh parsley
- ½ cup raw cashews
- 1 tablespoon fresh lemon juice
- ¼ teaspoon sea salt
- 1 tablespoon apple cider vinegar
- 2 tablespoons extra virgin olive oil

SALAD

- 6 Persian cucumbers (14 ounces), sliced
- 1 tablespoon black sesame seeds
- 2 sheets dried nori seaweed, slightly toasted, cut into 1-inch squares

Combine all the ingredients for the sauce except the oil in a blender and puree on high. Then slowly add the oil with the blender running on low speed. Blend until creamy. Coat the cucumbers with sauce and stir in the black sesame seeds. Sprinkle with nori and serve.

ROASTED ZUCCHINI SALAD

Serves 2

SALAD	DRESSING
2 medium zucchini, sliced	juice of ½ lemon
9 shiitake mushrooms, sliced thick	1 tablespoon rice wine vinegar
2 tablespoons extra virgin olive oil	2 tablespoons coconut yogurt
1 teaspoon sea salt	¼ teaspoon sea salt
1 teaspoon garlic powder	2 teaspoons raw honey
2–3 cups arugula leaves	1 tablespoon dried herb blend: chives,
6 basil leaves, chopped	dill, tarragon, chervil, white pepper
¼ cup raw pistachios	1 tablespoon olive oil

Preheat the oven to 375°F. Coat the zucchini and mushrooms with the olive oil. Sprinkle with sea salt and garlic powder. Spread the vegetables on a baking sheet and cook for 20 minutes, or until softened.

Combine all the dressing ingredients except the oil in a blender. Blend on high, then slowly add the oil with the blender running on low speed.

Place the arugula in bowls. Top with the basil, pistachios, and roasted zucchini and mushrooms. Add dressing to taste. Store remaining dressing in the refrigerator for up to one week.

FENNEL WILD RICE SALAD

Serves 1

SALAD	DRESSING
2 cups arugula leaves	¼ cup water
½ large fennel bulb, thinly sliced	¼ cup raw cashews
1 Persian cucumber, chopped (½ cup)	1 teaspoon miso paste
5 kalamata olives, pitted and chopped	1 tablespoon fresh tarragon
1 tablespoon capers, rinsed	¼ teaspoon sea salt
½ medium yellow bell pepper, chopped	¼ cup rice wine vinegar
½ cup cooked wild rice	

Toss all the salad ingredients together in a large bowl. Combine the dressing ingredients in a blender and blend until creamy. Toss the salad with the dressing and serve.

RICH SEAWEED SALAD

Serves 1 as an entree, 2 as a side dish

SALAD

- 3 cups chopped kale
- 2 tablespoons sauerkraut
- 12 cherry tomatoes, halved
- 8 kalamata olives, pitted and halved
- ½ medium avocado, peeled, pitted, and sliced
- 2 celery ribs, chopped
- ¼ cup dried, toasted nori, slightly toasted, cut into 1-inch squares
- 1 tablespoon black sesame seeds

LEMON CREAM VINAIGRETTE

- 1 tablespoon tahini
- juice of ½ medium lemon
- 2 tablespoons champagne vinegar
- ⅛ teaspoon sea salt
- 2 tablespoons extra virgin olive oil

Toss all the salad ingredients except the nori and sesame seeds together in a large bowl. Combine all the dressing ingredients except the oil in a blender and puree on high. Slowly add the oil with the blender running on low speed. Toss the salad with the dressing, then top with the nori and sesame seeds.

ROASTED BLACK PLUM AND FENNEL SALAD

Serves 1 as an entree, 2 as a side dish

SALAD

- 1 Japanese cucumber, diced (½ cup)
- ½ cup chopped radicchio
- 1 cup arugula leaves
- ¼ cup raw walnuts, soaked for 3 hours
- ⅓ cup cooked quinoa

ROASTED PLUM AND FENNEL

- 2 black plums, halved and pitted
- 1 medium fennel bulb, thinly sliced
- 1–2 tablespoons extra virgin olive oil

DRESSING

- 1 garlic clove, roasted (400°F for 10 minutes)
- 2 tablespoons balsamic vinegar
- 1 tablespoon rice wine vinegar
- 1 teaspoon raw honey
- ⅛ teaspoon sea salt
- 1 tablespoon minced fresh thyme
- 2 tablespoons extra virgin olive oil

Make the Salad: Toss all the ingredients together in a large bowl.

Make the Roasted Plum and Fennel: Preheat the oven to 450°F. Line a rimmed baking sheet with aluminum foil. Coat the plums and fennel in the olive oil, and spread on the prepared baking sheet. Roast for 10 minutes, until tender. Allow to cool.

Make the Dressing: Combine all the ingredients except the olive oil in a blender and blend on high. Reduce the speed to low and slowly add the oil.

Dish the salad into a bowl, then top with the roasted fennel and plums. Add dressing to taste. Store remaining dressing in the refrigerator for up to one week.

FRENCH HARICOTS VERTS SALAD

Serves 1

SALAD	DRESSING
2 cups arugula leaves	1 tablespoon minced fresh thyme
6 cherry tomatoes, halved	2 tablespoons red wine vinegar
½ medium field cucumber, peeled and chopped (½ cup)	1 tablespoon extra virgin olive oil
	1 teaspoon stone ground mustard
25 green beans (1 cup), trimmed and chopped	sea salt and black pepper, to taste
½ cup canned garbanzo beans, drained and rinsed	

Toss all the salad ingredients together in a large bowl. In a small bowl, whisk together all the dressing ingredients. Toss the salad with the dressing and serve.

CORN AND ARUGULA SUMMER SALAD

Serves 1

SALAD	DRESSING
kernels from 1 ear raw corn	¼ teaspoon sea salt
2 cups arugula leaves	1 tablespoon extra virgin olive oil
6 cherry tomatoes, halved	1½ teaspoons stone ground mustard
1 tablespoon minced fresh thyme	2 tablespoons rice wine vinegar
¼ cup cooked black rice	¼ teaspoon garlic powder
1 Japanese cucumber, chopped (½ cup)	1 tablespoon juice from freshly squeezed orange

Toss all the salad ingredients together in a large bowl. In a small bowl, whisk together all the dressing ingredients. Toss the salad with the dressing and serve.

GREEN CLEANSING SALAD

Serves 1

SALAD

10 asparagus spears
⅓ cup peas·
½ cup chopped fresh parsley
1 cup arugula leaves
¼ cup cooked quinoa
1 tablespoon raw pine nuts
15 mint leaves, minced

CITRUS VINAIGRETTE DRESSING

1½ teaspoons juice from freshly
  squeezed lime
1½ teaspoons juice from freshly
  squeezed orange
1 tablespoon minced shallot
1 tablespoon extra virgin olive oil
1 tablespoon apple cider vinegar
1 teaspoon tahini
1 teaspoon stone ground mustard
pinch of sea salt

Fill the bottom half of a steamer with water and bring to a boil. Prepare an ice bath by filling a bowl with ice water. Trim the ends off the asparagus spears and place the spears in the top half of the steamer pan. Then add the peas. Steam for 5 to 10 minutes depending on the thickness of the asparagus, or until the asparagus is tender. Then plunge into the ice bath to retain the color. Once the asparagus is cool to the touch, cut the spears into pieces and set aside to cool completely.

Toss all the salad ingredients except the pine nuts and mint together in a large bowl. In a small bowl, whisk together all the dressing ingredients. Toss the salad with the dressing, top with pine nuts and mint, and serve.

WILD RICE SALAD

Serves 2

SALAD	DRESSING
1 cup cooked peas	1 tablespoon juice from freshly squeezed lime
1 large tomato, diced	4 tablespoons extra virgin olive oil
6 shiitake mushrooms, chopped	¼ cup raw pine nuts
1 medium red, orange, or yellow bell pepper, chopped	1 tablespoon raw honey
¼ cup chopped cilantro	1 ½ teaspoons honey mustard
1 cup cooked wild rice	2 teaspoons finely chopped chives
	1 teaspoon sea salt
	1 teaspoon black pepper

Toss all the salad ingredients together in a large bowl. In a small bowl, whisk together all the dressing ingredients. Toss the salad with the dressing and serve.

BRUSSELS SPROUTS SALAD WITH PARSLEY LEMON VINAIGRETTE

Serves 1 as an entree, 2 as a side dish

SALAD	DRESSING
2 cups shaved brussels sprouts	1 tablespoon raw honey
1 cup chopped raw green beans	1 tablespoon minced fresh parsley
¼ cup dried cherries	1 ½ teaspoons red wine vinegar
¼ cup whole raw hazelnuts	1 tablespoon juice from freshly squeezed lemon (Meyer lemon is ideal)
	1 teaspoon grated lemon zest (Meyer lemon is ideal)
	1 ½ teaspoons Dijon mustard
	1 garlic clove, minced
	¼ cup extra virgin olive oil
	½ teaspoon sea salt
	black pepper to taste

Toss all the salad ingredients together in a large bowl. In a small bowl, whisk together all the dressing ingredients. Toss the salad with the dressing and serve.

CHINESE TEMPEH SALAD

Serves 2

SALAD

2–3 tablespoons coconut oil

3–4 ounces tempeh, sliced into thin pieces

½ medium eggplant, cut into small cubes

1 tablespoon miso paste

1 tablespoon ginger, peeled and minced

1 tablespoon brown rice vinegar

2 cups arugula leaves

1 seedless mandarin orange, separated into wedges

1 large carrot, peeled and finely sliced

½ medium head napa cabbage, thinly sliced

2 tablespoons finely chopped green onion

¼ cup sliced raw almonds

2 teaspoons black seasme seeds, for garnish

sea salt, to taste

DRESSING

4 tablespoons brown rice vinegar

3 tablespoons sesame oil

1 teaspoon ginger, peeled and minced

1 tablespoon black sesame seeds

2 teaspoons raw honey

Make the Salad: Heat the coconut oil in a large skillet over medium-low heat. Add the tempeh and eggplant, and cook for 5 minutes. Then stir in the miso, ginger, and brown rice vinegar. Make sure the eggplant and tempeh are coated. Sauté until soft, about 15 minutes, stirring frequently to make sure that the mixture does not burn. Remove from the pan and set aside to cool.

Place the arugula, mandarin orange, carrot, and cabbage in a large bowl. Add the sautéed eggplant and tempeh.

Make the Dressing: Combine all the ingredients into a blender or food processor. Blend until creamy.

Toss the salad with the dressing. Transfer to serving plates and top with green onion, almonds, and sesame seeds. Season with sea salt.

ASIAN ASPARAGUS SALAD

Serves 1 as an entree, 2 as a side dish

SALAD	DRESSING
15 asparagus spears, thinly sliced	1 garlic clove, minced
3 cups kale	1 tablespoon minced fresh ginger
¼ cup raw cashews	juice of 1 lime
1½ cups sliced snap peas	1 tablespoon raw honey
	1 tablespoon rice vinegar
	1 tablespoon coconut oil
	2 tablespoons extra virgin olive oil

Toss all the salad ingredients together in a large bowl. In a small bowl, whisk together all the dressing ingredients. Toss the salad with the dressing and serve.

SUMMER ASPARAGUS SALAD

Serves 1 as an entree, 2 as a side dish

SALAD

- 2 red or golden beets, peeled and sliced in ¼-inch rounds
- 1–2 tablespoons extra virgin olive oil
- 1 cup arugula leaves
- 1 cup chopped raw medium broccoli
- 1 medium avocado, peeled, pitted, and cubed
- 12 asparagus spears
- 3 tablespoons raw pistachios

DRESSING

- ½ teaspoon minced shallot
- 1½ teaspoons juice from freshly squeezed lemon
- 2 tablespoons white wine
- 1 teaspoon lemon zest
- 1½ teaspoons Dijon mustard
- ⅓ cup extra virgin olive oil
- 1 teaspoon raw honey

Make the Salad: Preheat the oven to 400°F. Place the beets on a rimmed baking sheet and toss with the olive oil. Roast for 35 to 40 minutes, or until tender. Allow to cool.

Fill the bottom half of a steamer with water and bring to a boil. Prepare an ice bath by filling a bowl with ice water. Trim the ends off the asparagus spears and place the spears in the top half of the steamer pan. Steam for 5 to 10 minutes depending on the thickness of the asparagus, or until the asparagus is tender. Then plunge into the ice bath to retain the color. Once the asparagus is cool to the touch, cut the spears into pieces and set aside to cool completely.

Layer the arugula, broccoli, avocado, and asparagus in a large bowl. Then top with the roasted beets and pistachios.

Make the dressing: Whisk all the ingredients in a small bowl, or puree in a blender. Drizzle over the salad and serve.

NORDIC HARVEST SALAD WITH LEMONY DRESSING AND SUPERFOODS

Serves 4

This beautiful recipe is the creation of a friend and talented health blogger, Elenore Bendel Zahn. She is a master of delicious recipes and everything health conscious, so it is no wonder she has made a presence in this book. Plus, she now makes a delicious product called the Nordic Superfood Mix, which contains tons of kidney superfoods. Please check out her website, www.earthsprout.com, for more recipes and inspiration. If you don't have Nordic Superfood Mix on hand, use other superfoods such as pomegranate seeds, mulberries, goldenberries, goji berries, raw pine nuts, and dried blueberries.

SALAD	LEMON-HONEY DRESSING
2 pounds brussels sprouts	1 tablespoon raw honey
2 teaspoons extra virgin coconut oil	4 tablespoons water
pinch of sea salt	3 tablespoons tahini
3 apples, thinly sliced	grated zest and juice of ½ lemon
3 cups arugula	pinch of sea salt
2 teaspoons Nordic Superfood Mix (to sprinkle over the dish when it's ready)	

Make the Salad: Preheat the oven to 400°F. Soak the brussels sprouts for 5 minutes in cold water to get rid of any sand or dirt in the leaves. Rinse thoroughly and cut off their stems with a small knife (careful— you do not want to cut too much and have the leaves fall off). Cut any large ones in half. Spread the brussels sprouts in a baking pan and toss with the coconut oil. Bake for 35 minutes (You want the cores of the sprouts to be a bit hard). Remove from the oven to cool.

Make the Lemon-Honey Dressing: Combine all the ingredients in a blender and puree, or whisk in a medium bowl until thoroughly combined.

Assemble the Salad: Mix the brussels sprouts, apple, and arugula in a large bowl. Drizzle the dressing over the salad and eat it as is, or serve with steamy hot quinoa or millet and freshly cracked black pepper. Top with Nordic superfood mix or other superfoods. This will give the dish that final nutritional punch.

Guidelines for making a killer salad

Start by choosing a green base (1 or more of the following):
- romaine lettuce
- kale (I like dinosaur kale, also called Lacinato or Tuscan kale)
- spinach
- chopped cabbage
- arugula
- butter lettuce

Add nutrient-boosting vegetables (choose 2 to 4 of the following):
- broccoli (raw or steamed)
- cabbage (if not used as a salad base)
- cucumber
- green beans (raw or steamed)
- celery
- mushrooms (button or shiitake are best)
- beets
- zucchini or other summer squash
- (raw or cooked)
- carrot
- bell pepper (green, red, orange or yellow; roasted or raw)
- tomato
- onion (red, sweet, or green)
- brussels sprouts (roasted or raw)
- fresh herbs (parsley, cilantro, tarragon, thyme, mint, dill, oregano)

Add a healthy fat (choose 1 or 2 of the following):
- olives
- avocado
- hemp seeds
- chia seeds
- raw nuts or seeds (walnut, pine nut, pistachio, cashew, almond, pumpkin, sunflower, flaxseed)

Add some bulk (choose 1 or 2 of the following):
- beans/legumes (kidney bean, cannellini bean, black bean, garbanzo bean, mung bean, lentil, lima bean)
- grains (buckwheat, quinoa, black rice, jasmine rice, brown rice, millet)

Optional: Add some odds and ends (choose 1 or 2 of the following):
- capers
- sauerkraut
- kimchi
- seaweed
- artichoke hearts
- nutritional yeast
- sun-dried tomatoes

Add a dressing (choose 1 of the following blends):
- Lemon juice, extra virgin olive oil, and sea salt
- Balsamic vinegar, olive oil, dried basil, black pepper, and sea salt
- Red wine vinegar, olive oil, sea salt, and Dijon mustard
- Rice wine vinegar, sesame oil, sea salt, and ginger
- Rice wine vinegar, coconut aminos (raw, gluten-free, soy sauce replacement), miso paste, and sesame oil
- Champagne vinegar, freshly squeezed orange juice, olive oil, crushed garlic, and sea salt
- Apple cider vinegar, Dijon mustard, garlic, sea salt, olive oil, chives, and thyme
- White wine vinegar, honey, olive oil, sea salt, tarragon, and chives

ENTREES

TAHINI, GOJI BERRY, AND KALE SALAD WITH WARM BHUTANESE BLACK RICE

Serves 1

SALAD

- 1 bunch kale, de-stemmed and thinly chopped (1 cup)
- 1 tablespoon juice from a freshly squeezed lemon
- 1 ounce dried goji berries
- 4 tablespoons raw pumpkin seeds
- 1½ cups cooked Bhutanese black rice

DRESSING

- 2 tablespoons tahini
- 1 teaspoon rice wine vinegar
- 1 teaspoon coconut aminos
- 1 teaspoon organic miso paste
- 1 teaspoon raw honey
- 1 tablespoon nutritional yeast
- ½ teaspoon sea salt
- ¼ teaspoon turmeric
- 1 tablespoon minced fresh thyme
- sea salt, to taste

Place the kale in a large bowl and add the lemon juice. Massage thoroughly with your fingers until the kale has reduced in size significantly and is soft, about 3 minutes.

In a blender or food processor, combine the ingredients for the dressing. Blend until creamy. Add the dressing to the kale and massage until the kale is fully coated. Mix in the goji berries and pumpkin seeds. Add salt to taste. Serve on top of warm, cooked rice.

RAW MARINARA AND KELP NOODLES

Serves 2

RAW MARINARA SAUCE

½ cup sun-dried tomatoes
½ cup chopped cherry tomatoes
1 tablespoon juice from a freshly
  squeezed lemon
1 tablespoon extra virgin olive oil
1 ½ teaspoons raw honey
1 tablespoon minced fresh basil
1 tablespoon minced fresh oregano
½ teaspoon sea salt
1 teaspoon minced garlic

NOODLES

1 (12-ounce) package kelp noodles
  (I like Sea Tangle; gluten-free
  buckwheat noodles — soba
  noodles — or zucchini noodles can
  be substituted for the kelp noodles)
1 teaspoon baking soda
2 cups water

TOPPINGS

2 tablespoons pitted and chopped
  kalamata olives
¼ cup chopped fresh basil
1 tablespoon nutritional yeast
  (optional)

Make the Raw Marinara Sauce: Combine the ingredients for the marinara sauce in a blender or food processor. Blend on high to puree. Set aside.

Make the Noodles: Soak the noodles in a large bowl with the baking soda and water for 20 minutes. Make sure they are completely submerged in the water. The baking soda will help soften them. When the noodles are done soaking, rinse them off, then top with raw marinara sauce, olives, and basil. Sprinkle with nutritional yeast, if desired.

POMEGRANATE EGGPLANT RATATOUILLE WITH CRISPY SAGE

Serves 4

CRISPY SAGE

20 fresh green sage leaves

1 tablespoon coconut oil

RATATOUILLE

2 tablespoons coconut oil, divided

2 garlic cloves, minced

1 small sweet onion, chopped

1 ½ pounds tomatoes, peeled and diced

1 teaspoon sea salt

1 medium eggplant, diced

1 medium zucchini, diced

1 large leek, washed, trimmed and sliced

1 jalapeño chile pepper, seeded and minced

3 tablespoons pomegranate molasses

3 tablespoons ketchup (free of high-fructose corn syrup)

1 tablespoon fennel seeds

black pepper and cayenne pepper, to taste

3 tablespoons chopped fresh parsley

Make the Crispy Sage: Wash the sage leaves and dry thoroughly. Line a plate with several layers of paper towels and set aside.

Warm the coconut oil in a small saucepan and heat over medium heat for 1 minute. Test the heat by adding one sage leaf to the oil. Make sure it fries in about 5 seconds. It should turn bright green, without browning. Once this happens, flip it over, and cook for another 5 seconds. If it does not turn green in 5 seconds or so, turn the heat up. If it browns too quickly, turn the heat down. Make sure there is enough oil to submerge the sage leaf. Once the leaf is bright green on both sides, place on the paper towels. Continue with the remaining sage leaves by adding four leaves at a time, frying on each side, and placing on the paper towels to cool.

Make the Ratatouille: Heat 1 tablespoon of the coconut oil over medium heat in a large skillet. Add the garlic and onion and cook, stirring, until translucent, about 5 minutes. Add the tomatoes and salt. Simmer, uncovered, for 10 to 15 minutes. Add the eggplant, zucchini, leek, jalapeño, molasses, and ketchup. Simmer, covered, for 20 to 30 minutes, until the vegetables are soft. Stir in the fennel seeds. Continue to simmer for about 5 minutes, until the flavors have blended. Add black pepper and cayenne. Top with the parsley and crispy sage.

MEDITERRANEAN QUINOA PASTA

Serves 2

8 ounces dry quinoa pasta (such as Ancient Harvest)

2 tablespoons extra virgin olive oil

½ medium onion, diced

2 garlic cloves, minced

1 tablespoon cumin seeds

¼ cup sun-dried tomatoes

2 tablespoons chopped fresh parsley

1 tablespoon minced fresh thyme

2 tablespoons raw pine nuts

sea salt and red chili pepper flakes, to taste

nutritional yeast (optional)

Cook the pasta according to package directions. Do not overcook; typically quinoa pasta needs 7 to 12 minutes.

In a medium skillet, heat the olive oil over low heat, then add the onion and garlic. Heat until translucent, stirring, about 5 minutes, and add the cumin. Stir for about 2 more minutes.

When the pasta is cooked, transfer it to a large bowl and stir in the sun-dried tomatoes, parsley, and thyme. Then drizzle on the onion, garlic, and cumin mixture. Divide into two bowls and top with pine nuts. Add salt and red chili flakes. Sprinkle with nutritional yeast, if desired.

ASIAN BLACK RICE WITH SWEET POTATO

Serves 2

1 tablespoon coconut oil
1 garlic clove, minced
1 tablespoon minced fresh ginger
½ cup minced sweet onion
½ cup diced sweet potato
½ cup diced red bell pepper
½ cup diced yellow summer squash
½ cup cooked black rice

1 teaspoon tamari or coconut aminos
juice of ½ lime
¼ teaspoon ground cumin
¼ teaspoon sea salt
1 teaspoon rice wine vinegar
¼ teaspoon turmeric
1 tablespoon pumpkin seeds

In a medium sauté pan or skillet, warm the coconut oil over medium heat. Add the garlic, ginger, and onion, and sauté until onion becomes iridescent, 5 to 10 minutes. Then add the sweet potato and cover the pan. Cook for about 20 minutes on medium heat, or until the sweet potato is softened but not completely cooked through. If necessary, add a little more coconut oil to prevent the potato from burning.

Add the bell pepper and squash. Cover again and cook until soft, about 10 minutes, then stir in the cooked black rice. Stir in the tamari or coconut aminos, lime juice, cumin, salt, rice wine vinegar, and turmeric. Top each serving with pumpkin seeds and serve.

SAGE SQUASH AND KALE BOWL

Serves 2

SAGE SQUASH

2 tablespoons coconut oil
½ teaspoon sea salt
3 tablespoons minced fresh sage
1 medium acorn squash, peeled and sliced into thin pieces

KALE SALAD

3 cups kale, chopped
¼ teaspoon sea salt
juice of ½ medium lemon
1 tablespoon tahini
1 tablespoon apple cider vinegar
1 tablespoon extra virgin olive oil
1 teaspoon raw honey
2 garlic cloves, minced
⅓ cup balsamic vinegar
½ cup toasted pumpkin seeds

Make the Sage Squash: Preheat the oven to 375°F. Mix the oil, salt, and sage in a small bowl. If the oil is still in a solid state, run under hot water to liquefy. Then coat the squash with the oil mixture. Arrange the squash pieces on a baking sheet and roast for 30 minutes. After the roasting time, turn on the oven's broiler and broil for 2 minutes. Set aside to cool.

Make the Kale Salad: Place the kale in a large bowl and add the salt and lemon juice. Massage with your fingers until the kale softens. Add the remaining ingredients, except the balsamic vinegar and pumpkin seeds, and massage in.

Make a balsamic reduction by heating the balsamic vinegar in a small saucepan over medium heat. Simmer slowly until it reduces by about half, stirring regularly to avoid burning the vinegar. Once it reduces to a thick syrup, 10 to 15 minutes, take it off the heat.

Assemble the Bowl: Add the roasted squash to the kale salad. Drizzle with the balsamic reduction and top with pumpkin seeds.

COLLARD WRAP WITH HAZELNUT PESTO

Serves 4

HAZELNUT PESTO

1 ½ cups basil leaves, chopped
1 cup parsley leaves, chopped
3 tablespoons fresh lemon juice
½ teaspoon sea salt
1 cup raw hazelnuts, soaked for 2 hours
1 garlic clove
⅓ cup extra virgin olive oil

COLLARD WRAP

4 collard greens leaves, including stems (larger leaves are best)
4 small tomatoes, sliced
2 medium avocados, peeled, pitted, and sliced
1 medium field cucumber, sliced
1 cup sprouts (any variety)

Make the Hazelnut Pesto: Combine all the ingredients in a blender or food processor and puree until smooth.

Make the Collard Wrap: Lay the collard leaves on a work surface. Spread pesto and top with tomato, avocado, cucumber, and sprouts. Wrap the collard leaves around the filling like a burrito and serve.

STUFFED SWEET POTATO

Serves 2

2 (6-ounce) sweet potatoes
1 tablespoon coconut oil
2 tablespoons tahini

¼ cup minced fresh parsley
¼ cup sauerkraut
sea salt and nutritional yeast, to taste

Preheat the oven to 375°F. Wash and scrub the sweet potatoes thoroughly, and rub them with the coconut oil. Place on a baking sheet and bake for about 45 minutes to 1 hour, or until cooked through.

Cut the baked sweet potatoes open and add the tahini, parsley, and sauerkraut. Sprinkle with sea salt and nutritional yeast.

ASIAN TEMPEH, KALE, AND BLACK RICE BOWL

Serves 4

1–2 tablespoons coconut oil
1 small sweet onion, chopped
4 garlic cloves, chopped
1 (8-ounce) package tempeh
3–4 cups chopped kale
juice from ½ medium lemon
1 tablespoon brown rice vinegar

1 tablespoon miso paste
1 tablespoon coconut aminos
pinch of red pepper flakes (optional)
3 cups cooked black rice
1 tablespoon minced, peeled ginger
sea salt, to taste

Warm the coconut oil in a large skillet over medium-high heat. Stir in the onion and garlic, and sauté until the onion softens a bit, 2 to 3 minutes. Stir in the tempeh and continue to sauté until it heats up and starts to brown. Stir in the kale. Cook the greens for 2 to 3 minutes, until they collapse and soften. You can put a lid on the pan for a couple of minutes to expedite the process.

Mix in the lemon juice, brown rice vinegar, miso, coconut aminos, and red pepper flakes, if using. You will have to thoroughly mix in the miso to prevent it from clumping. Add the cooked rice and sauté until hot, then add the ginger and sea salt.

BUTTERNUT SQUASH MARINARA

Serves 2

4 tablespoons olive oil, divided
1 large butternut squash (2 pounds), peeled
3–4 garlic cloves, minced
½ large onion, diced
3 medium carrots, peeled and chopped
1 large leek, washed, trimmed and chopped

3 celery ribs, chopped
1 (28-ounce) can tomato sauce
2 tablespoons minced fresh thyme
1 tablespoon minced fresh oregano
sea salt, to taste
pinch of nutritional yeast

Preheat the oven to 350°F and coat a baking dish or rimmed baking sheet with a little of the olive oil. Slice the butternut squash in half lengthwise and scoop out the seeds and strings. Then slice into moon-shaped pieces about ½ inch wide. Divide 1 tablespoon of the olive oil among the squash pieces and lightly coat, and arrange in the prepared dish. Bake for 25 to 40 minutes, until soft. Once cooked, remove from the oven and peel off the skin. Set aside the cooked squash and keep warm.

While the squash is cooking, in a large pot heat the remaining 3 table-spoons olive oil over medium-low heat, then add the garlic and onion. Cook for about 10 minutes, stirring frequently. Once the garlic and onion begin to soften, add the carrots, leek, and celery. Cook for about 10 minutes and then stir in the tomato sauce, thyme, and oregano. Cook for at least 15 minutes on low heat so that the flavors combine. This sauce is always better the longer you cook it, as the flavors infuse and become richer. Once the sauce is done, season with sea salt.

Serve the sauce over the butternut squash and sprinkle with nutritional yeast.

COCONUT CURLY CRISPY KALE

Serves 2

2 tablespoons coconut aminos

⅓ cup coconut oil

2 cups de-stemmed, chopped kale, in 1-inch squares

1½ cups unsweetened coconut flakes

½ teaspoon sea salt

2 cups cooked red rice

2 tablespoons raw pine nuts

3 tablespoons hemp seeds

Preheat the oven to 350°F. In a large bowl, whisk together the coconut aminos and coconut oil. If the oil is in a solid state, run the jar under hot water to liquefy. Combine the kale and coconut flakes in a large bowl. Add the oil-aminos mixture and toss well. Sprinkle with sea salt. Spread the kale across a rimmed baking sheet and bake for 12 to 20 minutes, until the kale is crispy. Make sure it does not burn.

Serve over warm, cooked red rice. Top with pine nuts and hemp seeds.

"CHEESY" COLLARD WRAPS

Serves 6

CASHEW PARMESAN

1 cup raw cashews

¼ cup nutritional yeast

1 tablespoon fresh lemon juice

1 teaspoon sea salt

pinch of black pepper

SUNFLOWER SEED CHEESE

⅓ cup lemon juice

½ cup coconut aminos

4 garlic cloves, minced (roast them if you prefer a lighter garlic taste)

2¾ cups raw sunflower seeds, ground to a fine powder in a food processor or coffee grinder

2–3 tablespoons finely chopped fresh dill or tarragon

1 teaspoon turmeric (optional)

COLLARD WRAP

12 collard greens leaves, including stems (larger leaves are best)

1 cup cherry tomatoes, halved

½ cup fresh herb blend: fresh tarragon, chives, and parsley, finely chopped

OPTIONAL TOPPINGS (PER WRAP)

1 tablespoon olives

1 tablespoon sun-dried tomatoes

¼ cup sprouts

1 tablespoon chopped cucumber

Make the Cashew Parmesan: Preheat the oven to 250°F. Spread the cashews on a baking dish and bake for 15 minutes. Keep an eye on them and stir if necessary to prevent burning. Put the cashews, nutritional yeast, lemon juice, salt, and pepper in a food processor or high-speed blender and process until ground into a chunky powder. Refrigerate leftovers in an airtight container for up to a week.

Make the Sunflower Seed Cheese: Combine all the ingredients in a food processor or high-speed blender and process until a smooth paste forms. Refrigerate leftovers in an airtight container for up to a week.

Make the Collard Wrap: Lay the collard leaves on a work surface. Spread sunflower cheese, then top with the tomatoes, herbs, and other desired toppings. Cover with cashew Parmesan. Wrap the collard leaves around the filling like a burrito and serve.

GARLICKY SWEET POTATO AND GREENS

Serves 2

1 tablespoon coconut oil
4 garlic cloves, finely diced
½ large sweet onion, finely chopped
1 large sweet potato, peeled and diced
½ medium head green cabbage, finely sliced
1 bunch (1 pound) collard greens, de-stemmed and thinly sliced

2 tablespoons extra virgin olive oil
sea salt and nutritional yeast, to taste

OPTIONAL TOPPINGS

1 tablespoon black sesame seeds
1 tablespoon coconut aminos
1 tablespoon rice wine vinegar

In a large skillet, warm the coconut oil over medium-low heat. Add the garlic and onion, and sauté for 5 to 10 minutes, or until the onion is translucent. Add the sweet potato and cabbage, stir to coat in the olive oil, and cover. If necessary, add a little extra coconut oil to make sure the vegetables do not burn. Cook for about 5 to 8 minutes. After the sweet potato and cabbage have begun to soften, add the collard greens. Cover and reduce the heat to low. Cook for another 15 minutes, or until the vegetables are soft.

Serve warm. Drizzle the olive oil over the top, and add sea salt and nutritional yeast. Add any or all of the optional ingredients, and toss together.

MEDITERRANEAN-STYLE POLENTA WITH WALNUT-ASPARAGUS PESTO

Serves 2–3

WALNUT-ASPARAGUS PESTO

25 stalks of asparagus, steamed
½ cup raw walnuts
½ cup basil, chopped
½ cup parsley, chopped
½ teaspoon sea salt
1 tablespoon juice from a freshly squeezed lemon
1 small jalapeño, minced
¼ cup extra virgin olive oil
1 clove garlic, minced

POLENTA

3 tablespoons coconut oil, divided
1 (18-ounce) tube precooked polenta, thickly sliced into ½-inch circles
1 large eggplant, thinly sliced into rounds
3 tablespoons finely chopped fresh rosemary
⅓ cup balsamic vinegar
½ cup walnut-asparagus pesto
1 cup sun-dried tomatoes, chopped (preserved in olive oil is best)
¼ cup finely chopped fresh basil
2 tablespoons kalamata olives, pitted and chopped
2 tablespoons roasted red pepper (from a jar), chopped
2 tablespoons pine nuts
sea salt to taste

Make the Walnut-Asparagus Pesto: Place ingredients in a blender or a food processor. Pulse until thick and chunky. Set aside.

Make the Polenta: Preheat the oven to 350°F.

Warm 1 tablespoon of the coconut oil in a large skillet over medium heat. Add slices of polenta. Cook the polenta until one side lightly browns, 5 to 10 minutes, then flip and cook the other side until lightly browned and slightly crispy, 5 to 10 minutes more. Once the polenta is done, remove from the skillet and place on a dish or cooling rack.

Coat the bottom of a rimmed baking sheet or glass baking dish with 1 tablespoon of the coconut oil and add the eggplant slices. Coat the top side of each eggplant slice with the remaining 1 tablespoon coconut oil and lightly sprinkle with salt and rosemary. Bake for about 20 minutes or until the eggplant is soft. Remove from the oven to cool.

Make a balsamic reduction by heating the balsamic vinegar in a small saucepan over medium heat. Simmer slowly until it reduces by about half, stirring regularly to avoid burning the vinegar. Once it reduces to a thick syrup, take it off the heat.

Assemble the components by creating a tower. Layer in this order: eggplant, polenta, walnut-asparagus pesto, sun-dried tomatoes, basil, olives, roasted pepper, and pine nuts. Drizzle balsamic vinegar reduction over the top.

INSIDE-OUT SUSHI BOWL

Serves 2

8 ounces tempeh

2 tablespoons miso paste

1 tablespoon fresh ginger, peeled and minced

juice of ½ medium lemon

2–3 tablespoons coconut aminos

2–3 tablespoons brown rice vinegar

1–2 tablespoons coconut oil

1 eggplant, chopped

2 cups cooked basmati rice

1 avocado, peeled, pitted, and sliced

2 tablespoons chopped fresh chives

1 sheet nori seaweed, slightly toasted, cut into 1-inch squares

3–4 tablespoons black sesame seeds

Slice the tempeh into four pieces widthwise. Whisk the miso and ginger together in a small bowl, then spread a layer of the mixture on one side of each tempeh slice. Combine the lemon juice, coconut aminos, and brown rice vinegar in a bowl or Ziploc bag. Add the tempeh and let marinate for up to 1 hour.

Warm the coconut oil in a large skillet over medium-low heat, then add the eggplant and cover. Sauté until soft, 15 to 20 minutes.

Remove the tempeh from the bag and reserve the marinade. In a second skillet, cook the tempeh. Turn the heat up to medium-high for about 5 minutes, or until the tempeh is browned on one side. Flip over and continue to cook until the tempeh is slightly browned and crispy. Be careful not to burn it by adding more oil if needed.

Scoop warm, cooked rice into individual bowls, and add the eggplant and tempeh. Top with avocado, chives, nori, and sesame seeds. Drizzle the reserved marinade over the bowls. If there is not enough left, feel free to make some more and add it.

PARSNIP SUSHI ROLLS

Serves 2

PARSNIP "RICE"

4 medium parsnips, peeled and chopped

1 tablespoon coconut aminos

1 tablespoon coconut oil

2 teaspoons brown rice vinegar

1 tablespoon miso paste

1 teaspoon sea salt

1 tablespoon wasabi powder (optional)

ROLLS

4 sheets raw nori seaweed

1 medium red bell pepper, sliced into thin strips

½ medium field cucumber, seeded and sliced lengthwise into thin strips (½ cup)

1 avocado, peeled, pitted, and thinly sliced

½ medium beet, peeled and sliced thin, and then vertically into long, thin strips

2 cups sprouts (any variety)

TOPPINGS

1 tablespoon black sesame seeds

2 tablespoons wasabi paste

4 ounces pickled ginger

4 ounces coconut aminos

fresh lemon juice (optional)

Make the Parsnip "Rice": Place all the ingredients in a food processor or high-speed blender, and pulse until the mixture takes on the consistency of rice.

Make the Rolls: Place a sheet of nori in a horizontal direction on your cutting board. Cover the bottom two-thirds of the sheet with an even layer of parsnip "rice." Fill the center with strips of bell pepper, cucumber, avocado, and beet, then top with sprouts. Roll up from the bottom of the sheet (the edge that has filling on it), and seal the end with a bit of water. I like to roll it as if it were rolling a sleeping bag or yoga mat, gently but tightly. Use a sharp knife to slice the sushi into even rolls. Be sure the knife is sharp, because if it is too dull it will pull the nori and wreck the shape of the roll.

Top with sesame seeds and serve with wasabi, ginger, and coconut aminos. Drizzle with lemon juice if desired.

Variations: Great additions or variations include mango, strawberries, raw seed or nut burger, kale, arugula, tomato, sun-dried tomato, and olives.

RED CURRY TEMPEH BOWL

Serves 2

4 small to medium Yukon Gold
    potatoes (1 pound), cut into chunks
1 tablespoon coconut oil
1 medium sweet onion, chopped
1 teaspoon cumin seeds
1 teaspoon sweet curry powder
¼ teaspoon turmeric

½ teaspoon cayenne pepper
1 teaspoon ground cinnamon
1 (14-ounce) can diced tomatoes
8 ounces tempeh, sliced widthwise
    into thin pieces
2 teaspoons sea salt

Bring a few inches of water to boil in a large pot. Place the potatoes in the pot, reduce the heat so the water is at a low boil, and cook for 15 to 20 minutes, or until the potatoes are soft.

Meanwhile, in a large skillet, warm the coconut oil over medium-low heat. Add the onion and cook for about 5 minutes, stirring, until soft. Stir in the cumin, curry, turmeric, cayenne, cinnamon, and tomatoes. Cook for about 10 minutes on low heat until all the flavors have blended. Then transfer to a high-speed blender or food processor and blend until smooth.

Transfer the sauce back to the skillet and add the cooked potatoes and tempeh. Stir together and cook for another 5 minutes. Stir in the salt and serve warm.

SIDE DISHES AND SNACKS

POMEGRANATE PERSIAN KALE CHIPS

Serves 3

1 cup raw walnuts

3 large roasted red bell peppers (from a jar is okay)

1 tablespoon pomegranate molasses

1 tablespoon extra virgin olive oil

3 garlic cloves, minced

1 tablespoon juice from a freshly squeezed lemon

1 teaspoon ground cumin

½ teaspoon sea salt

½ teaspoon ground cinnamon

2 large bunches kale, de-stemmed and cut into 1-inch squares

Place all ingredients except the kale in a food processor or blender and blend until creamy. Place the kale pieces in a large bowl and pour the cream sauce on top. Massage the sauce into the kale with your fingers, until kale softens, about 3 minutes.

If using an oven, preheat it to 350°F and line a rimmed baking sheet with parchment paper. Spread the kale chips on the prepared sheet and bake for 10 minutes, or until crispy. Make sure to check frequently so that they do not burn. You may have to stir to prevent burning.

If using a dehydrator, lay the kale chips on the sheets and turn the dehydrator to 125°F. Let the chips dehydrate for 6 hours, or until crispy. Of you want to make them "raw," dehydrate at 110°F for about 10 hours.

ZUCCHINI "HUMMUS" WITH HOMEMADE GLUTEN-FREE CRACKERS

Serves 3

ZUCCHINI HUMMUS

2 cups raw almonds, soaked for 3 hours

2 large zucchini, chopped (about 3 cups)

3 tablespoons tahini

3 tablespoons extra virgin olive oil

2 tablespoons juice from a freshly squeezed lemon

2 teaspoons sea salt

2 teaspoons ground cumin

1 teaspoon paprika

1 teaspoon garlic powder

CRACKERS

1 cup almond flour

3 tablespoons hemp seeds

1 tablespoon nutritional yeast

1 tablespoon tomato powder

½ teaspoon garlic powder

½ teaspoon sea salt

¼ teaspoon baking soda

3 tablespoons extra virgin olive oil

1 tablespoon minced fresh basil

1½ teaspoons minced fresh thyme

1½ teaspoons minced fresh oregano

1½ teaspoons minced fresh rosemary

1½ teaspoons black sesame seeds

Make the Zucchini "Hummus": Blend all the ingredients in a high-speed blender or food processor until thick, like hummus.

Make the Crackers: Preheat the oven to 350°F and line a rimmed baking sheet with parchment paper. Mix the ingredients together in a large bowl. Spread the "dough" on the prepared baking sheet evenly, smoothing out any clumps. Bake for 10 to 18 minutes. Make sure to check frequently, because the crackers cook quickly and you don't want them to burn.

Serve the crackers with zucchini hummus.

EGGLESS EGG SALAD

This "egg" salad can be eaten on its own, in a salad, with gluten-free crackers, or as a filling for collard greens wraps.

Serves 4

MUSTARD "MAYO"

- ½ cup coconut water
- 2 garlic cloves, minced
- 1 tablespoon juice from freshly squeezed lemon
- 1 tablespoon mustard powder
- ½ teaspoon sea salt
- 1 cup raw cashews, soaked for 3 hours
- ½ teaspoon turmeric
- 1 tablespoon apple cider vinegar

SALAD

- meat of 1 coconut, diced into small cubes
- ½ medium fennel bulb, diced
- 2 celery ribs, diced
- 3 tablespoons chopped cilantro
- ¼ cup raw pine nuts
- 2 teaspoons paprika

Make the Mustard "Mayo": Blend all the ingredients in a high-speed blender or food processor until smooth.

Make the Salad: Mix the coconut, fennel, celery, and cilantro together in a large bowl. Toss the salad with the mustard "mayo," then top with the pine nuts and paprika.

"CHEESY" BROCCOLI

Serves 2

2 cups chopped broccoli
1 tablespoon coconut oil
½ medium sweet onion, minced
2 garlic cloves, minced
1–2 tablespoons extra virgin olive oil
3 tablespoons nutritional yeast
1 tablespoon red wine vinegar

¼ teaspoon sea salt
1 tablespoon tahini
1 tablespoon minced fresh dill
2 tablespoons capers, rinsed
2 tablespoons sun-dried tomatoes
black pepper, to taste

Bring 1 inch of water to boil over high heat in a saucepan with a steamer. Add the broccoli to the steamer, reduce the heat to medium, and cover. Cook for 5 minutes, or until the broccoli is soft. Remove from the heat and set aside to cool.

Warm the coconut oil in a small sauté pan or skillet over medium heat Add the onion and garlic, and sauté until onion is translucent, about 5 minutes. Transfer the onion and garlic to a large bowl. Add the olive oil, nutritional yeast, red wine vinegar, salt, and tahini. Mix thoroughly with your hands. Add the dill, capers, and sun-dried tomatoes, and mix again. Then toss in the steamed broccoli. Make sure to mix gently to avoid breaking apart the broccoli. Season with pepper.

RAW MEDITERRANEAN CAULIFLOWER

Serves 4

1 large head cauliflower
1 tablespoon extra virgin olive oil
1 tablespoon red wine vinegar
1 tablespoon prepared horseradish
juice of ½ medium lemon

1 teaspoon sea salt
½ cup finely chopped fresh parsley
2 tablespoons finely chopped fresh mint
1 medium red bell pepper, diced
1 large tomato, diced

Cut off the bottom of the cauliflower below the florets and remove the leaves. Cut in half and separate the florets. Place the cauliflower, olive oil, red wine vinegar, horseradish, lemon juice, salt, parsley, and mint in a food processor. Pulse 4 or 5 times, just until the mixture is the consistency of rice. Don't pulse too much or you'll end up with cauliflower mush. Transfer to a large bowl and toss with the bell pepper and tomato.

To make into a meal, add cauliflower to a grain such as quinoa, or lima or cannellini beans.

WALNUT-ASPARAGUS PESTO CAPRESE

Serves 4

25 asparagus spears, lightly steamed
½ cup raw walnuts
½ cup chopped fresh basil
½ cup chopped fresh parsley
½ teaspoon sea salt
1 tablespoon lemon juice

1 small jalapeño chile pepper, seeded and minced
¼ cup extra virgin olive oil
1 garlic clove, chopped
2 large tomatoes, thickly sliced
6 basil leaves, chopped
truffle oil (optional)

Bring 1 inch of water to boil over high heat in to a large pot with a steamer. Prepare an ice bath by filling a bowl with ice water. Add the asparagus to the boiling water and reduce the heat to medium. Cover and cook for 5 to 10 minutes, or until the asparagus is tender. Once cooked, plunge into the ice bath. Submerge, then remove from the water. Set aside.

To make the pesto, place all the remaining ingredients except the tomatoes, basil, and truffle oil in a blender or a food processor, and pulse until thick and chunky. Cover each tomato slice with a dollop of pesto. Then top with basil and truffle oil, if using.

CAULIFLOWER CREAM PUREE

Serves 2

1 medium to large head cauliflower, cut into florets
1 tablespoon coconut oil
½ medium sweet or yellow onion, chopped
2 garlic cloves, minced

1 tablespoon minced fresh rosemary
2 tablespoons prepared horseradish (1½ tablespoons for less spice)
½ teaspoon sea salt
2 tablespoons unsweetened almond milk, or more as needed

Bring about 1 inch of water to a boil in the bottom of a large pot. Place a steamer basket in the pot and add the cauliflower florets, and cover. Steam until tender, 5 to 8 minutes, then remove from the heat.

Warm the coconut oil in a large sauté pan or skillet over medium heat. Add the onion and garlic, and sauté for about 5 minutes, or until the onion is translucent. Transfer the garlic and onions to a blender or food processor. Add the steamed cauliflower, rosemary, horseradish, salt, and almond milk. Puree until creamy. For a thinner consistency, add more almond milk.

This dish can be served as a side dish or snack. You can also pour it over a grain, beans, or steamed vegetables to make a complete meal.

BLACK CHERRY CHIA PUDDING

Serves 2

4 tablespoons chia seeds
1 cup pitted black cherries
⅓ cup unsweetened almond milk
½ teaspoon vanilla extract

TOPPINGS

2 tablespoons hemp seeds
2 tablespoons raw walnut pieces
2 tablespoons raw honey or molasses (optional)

Combine the chia seeds, cherries, almond milk, and vanilla in a blender. Blend until thick and creamy. Transfer to a bowl, cover, and refrigerate overnight to thicken.

You can add more almond milk if you want to thin the pudding, or if it's too thin, add more chia seeds to thicken it. Top with hemp seeds and walnut pieces. If you want to sweeten it, add a little raw honey or molasses.

BANANA VANILLA AVOCADO PUDDING

Serves 2

2 medium avocados, peeled, pitted, and sliced

2 tablespoons raw honey

2½ teaspoons vanilla extract

2 medium, ripe bananas

2 tablespoons full-fat coconut milk (from a can)

TOPPINGS

2 tablespoons unsweetened shredded coconut

2 tablespoons sliced almonds

Combine the avocados, honey, vanilla, bananas, and coconut milk in a blender or food processor. Blend until thick and creamy. Top with coconut shreds and sliced almonds, if desired.

ANTIOXIDANT-RICH CHIA PUDDING

Serves 2

⅓ cup chia seeds

1 cup fresh or frozen and thawed cranberries

1 cup coconut water

8 dates, pitted

1 teaspoon vanilla extract

2 tablespoons pomegranate seeds

¼ cup raw cashews, soaked for 3 hours

2 drops stevia, 1 tablespoon raw honey, or 1 tablespoon grade-B or #2 maple syrup (optional, to sweeten)

Combine the chia seeds, cranberries, coconut water, dates, and vanilla extract in a blender. Blend until thick and creamy. You can add more coconut water if you want to thin it, or if it's too thin, add more chia seeds to thicken it. Transfer to a bowl, cover, and refrigerate overnight to thicken.

In the morning, remove the pudding from the refrigerator and top it with pomegranate seeds and cashews. If desired, add stevia, honey, or maple syrup to sweeten the pudding.

APRICOT CHIA BOWL

Serves 1

3 apricots, pitted

2 tablespoons chia seeds

1 tablespoon raw honey

1 teaspoon vanilla extract

½ cup coconut water or unsweetened almond milk

TOPPINGS

1 teaspoon hemp seeds

1 teaspoon bee pollen

1 teaspoon dried blueberries

1 teaspoon raw walnut pieces

Combine the apricots, chia seeds, honey, vanilla, and coconut water or almond milk in a blender. Blend until the apricots are pureed and the consistency is smooth. Transfer to a bowl and refrigerate overnight.

In the morning, top with hemp seeds, bee pollen, dried blueberries, and walnut pieces, before serving.

"FRENCH FRIES" WITH THE WORKS

Serves 3

SWEET POTATO FRIES

3 tablespoons coconut oil, divided

3 (6-ounce) sweet potatoes, cut into french fries

¼ teaspoon sea salt

"CHEESY MAYO"

2 cups raw almonds

¼ cup extra virgin olive oil

5 tablespoons juice from a freshly squeezed lemon

1 tablespoon nutritional yeast

1 teaspoon sea salt

½ cup purified water

CARAMELIZED ONION

1 tablespoon coconut oil or ghee

1 medium sweet onion, chopped

SECRET SAUCE

½ cup "Cheesy Mayo"

1 tablespoon ketchup (free of high-fructose corn syrup)

1 tablespoon relish (free of high-fructose corn syrup)

Make the Sweet Potato Fries: Preheat the oven to 375°F and grease a rimmed baking sheet with 1 tablespoon of the coconut oil. Toss the cut sweet potatoes in the remaining 2 tablespoons of the coconut oil and the salt. If the oil is in a solid state, run the jar under hot water until it liquefies. Evenly spread out the sweet potatoes on the baking sheet. Bake for 20 minutes, then flip the fries to prevent burning. Bake for another 20 minutes, or until crispy. Remove from the oven to cool.

Make the "Cheesy Mayo": Combine all the ingredients in a food processor or high-speed blender and blend until smooth.

Make the Caramelized Onion: In a skillet large enough to fit the onion comfortably, heat the oil or ghee over medium-high heat, until the oil shimmers. Then add the onion, stirring to coat it in the oil. Spread the onion out evenly across the pan and let it cook, stirring occasionally. Depending on your stovetop burner, you may need to reduce the heat to medium or medium-low to prevent the onion from burning or drying out. Cook for 20 to 30 minutes, or until the onion has caramelized to a nice brown color. Be sure to stir throughout the process to prevent burning, but don't stir too often or the onion won't brown. When caramelized, set aside.

Make the Secret Sauce: Stir together the "Cheesy Mayo," ketchup, and relish until well combined. This ratio makes about ½ cup, but you can make more or less depending on how "saucy" you want your fries.

Fill a plate or bowl with the sweet potato fries, then top with secret sauce and caramelized onion.

CHAPTER ELEVEN

FAQS

Now that you made your way this far, I know you are dying to ask questions. Am I right? I have included every single question I could think of, along with my best attempts at complete answers. It is quite possible that I left out your particular question, and if this is the case I urge you to consult your doctor or alternative practitioner for more information.

Q. I have a medical condition. Is performing the kidney cleanse safe?
A. In all cases of disease or a diagnosed dysfunction, you must consult your doctor before performing the kidney cleanse. Changing your diet or taking supplements can alter your biochemistry, so it is imperative to discuss your particular condition before moving forward.

I also refer you to the chapter "Special Programs" on page 123, which contains many modifications to the kidney cleanse that you can review with your doctor. While some people may not be able to take the herbs or undergo the juice feast, they can usually follow the diet, especially if they pair it with the food restrictions suggested for various kidney conditions.

Q. Is it safe to do the cleanse while I am pregnant or breastfeeding?
A. I never recommend undergoing a cleanse of any kind when you are pregnant or breastfeeding because moving toxins in your body may be harmful to the baby. On the other hand, you most likely will be able to follow the kidney cleanse food plan in addition to adding some of the kidney cleanse juices to your diet, but I do not suggest juice feasting. You should discuss the use of supplements and herbs with your doctor.

Q. Will I get side effects from detoxification?
A. Every person is different. Some feel amazing the whole time, and others go through a period in which they experience symptoms such as fatigue, a runny or congested nose, headaches, a foggy head, or trouble concentrating. These are all normal reactions and they should pass, especially if you are

following the recommendations for adjunct therapies and supplements, and drinking plenty of water. If symptoms do not subside, or become troublesome or severe, please contact your doctor without delay.

Q. Will I lose weight on this cleanse?

A. When your body comes into balance by reducing its toxic load and improving its metabolic processes, it will shed unhealthy toxic weight. Excess fat stored in the body is simply a defense mechanism to protect the body from toxins, and when the toxins are cleared the body has no further use for that fat. This cleanse also focuses on incorporating healthy, nutrient-dense foods known to increase metabolism, balance hormones naturally, and promote normal bowel eliminations, thereby leading to a healthy weight. In addition, you will be exercising, using stress-reduction techniques, and getting plenty of rest, all of which promote a healthy weight. However, if you are underweight, the juice feast may not be a good idea for you. Talk to your doctor before proceeding.

Q. I take pharmaceutical drugs. Will they interact with the herbs? Should I stop my medications?

A. Always discuss possible interactions with your doctor before taking any supplements or herbs.

You should never modify your medications without talking to your doctor. However, any cleanse or change in diet can improve the way your body functions, which may reduce your dosage. I recommend that you have your doctor monitor your dosage carefully.

Q. I am currently taking supplements. Should I continue taking them on the cleanse?

A. If you are taking supplements as part of a program designed for you by a practitioner, then please check with that person to find out if it is okay to continue taking them. If you are taking supplements for general nutrition (essential fatty acids, vitamin D, minerals, antioxidants) and digestion that you have chosen on your own, you can stay on those as well. The only supplements that I suggest eliminating are detoxifiers or anti-infectives (to prevent infection). These supplements may push too many toxins through the system and overload the kidneys, reducing the effectiveness of the cleansing program.

Q. Can I do the cleanse if I choose not to use the recommended supplements?
A. Yes. While the supplements are included to aid in the detoxification process and to help you feel your best during your cleanse, they are not required. However, I do recommend that you use them. They are intended to minimize any detoxification reactions such as headaches, poor mood, and fatigue, and they support kidney function and repair, making the cleanse much more effective. If you are dedicating yourself to a month-long cleanse, why not go for the gold?

Q. I noticed that the herbs and foods used in the cleanse are diuretics. How do diuretics help to cleanse the kidney?
A. Diuretics increase the production of urine. They are used in cleansing the kidneys because they assist in the passage of waste products that otherwise may remain stagnant in the kidney, causing damage, inflammation, and possibly stones. In addition, they help to balance the minerals in the kidneys.

Q. I have heard that herbs can be toxic to the kidneys, especially since they are not standardized and proper labeling is not enforced. How can I know they are safe?
A. Many companies do not comply with general health standards, selling products that may contain heavy metals such as mercury, arsenic, cadmium, and lead, as well as other toxins. Just because a supplement or herb says "natural" and is sold in a health food store does not mean it is safe. I am very aware of this concern, and having worked for a supplement manufacturer, I understand the risks and know what questions to ask. All the supplements and herbs that I recommend in this book have been scrutinized for quality and safety. I urge you to follow my recommendations and to use only the supplements recommended to you by a licensed practitioner. The companies I trust are run like pharmaceutical firms, complying with standards such as NSF (an independent certifying agency) and GMP (Good Manufacturing Practices). It is important to be informed about all the supplements and medications you are taking.

I also want to assure you that I chose herbs and supplements proven the safest for the kidneys, even for people with kidney disease. Many of the kidney cleansing herbs and formulas on the market contain substances that have been shown to be toxic to the kidneys. As always, consult your doctor before taking any supplements.

Q. I have issues with my blood sugar (hypo or hyperglycemia). Is it safe for me to do the juice feast?

A. Juice feasting can produce many long-term benefits, but you must be careful since it can affect your blood sugar in the short term. I recommend that you avoid any juices high in sugar (those containing carrots, beets, or fruit), and focus on green juices. I would also suggest adding protein in the form of protein powders, nut milks, and/or blue green algae into the daily regime during the cleanse. Adding a small amount of oil such as flax, olive, hemp, or borage may help balance blood sugar as well. Remember to consult your doctor before proceeding.

Q. Will I feel as if I'm starving during the juice feast?

A. The juice feast is not intended to starve the body but rather to supply it with beneficial nutrients. You may feel hungry at times, but it will pass. Many people actually even feel full from all the juice and can't finish the recommended amount. Everyone is different. Much of this process is mental — your body is reacting to the fear of starvation and not to a lack of nutrients.

Q. Can I drink more or less than the recommended amount of juice during the juice feast?

A. Absolutely. The juice plan is merely a recommendation. Feel free to drink as much or as little as you like, but make sure you consume enough to provide the nutrients your body needs to detoxify and repair. Typically four or five juices a day is sufficient.

Q. Should I juice everything all at once for the day? How about for all 3 days?

A. Once you juice your vegetables and fruits, the nutrition and enzyme content begins to degrade unless you are using a hydraulic press juicer. I suggest making your juice right before you drink it. If that is not possible, you can juice everything for the day and keep it refrigerated.

Making the juice for the 3-day feast all at once is not ideal. Just as you wouldn't want to eat 3-day-old food, you don't want to drink 3-day-old juice. If you will not be able to do the feast without making all the juice in advance, then go ahead. Better to do the 3-day feast than not, even if you are drinking old juice. Once again, the exception is juice made with a hydraulic press juicer—it will last pretty well for 3 days.

Q. Can I use bottled juice from the market?

A. No. Store-bought juice is full of sugar and is not a living food. It is often made from concentrates, produced months earlier, and pasteurized. The only exception is juice purchased from a vendor that makes it fresh. For example, juice bars and some health food stores (such as many Whole Foods locations) and cafés make juice fresh.

Q. What if I need to eat something during the juice feast?

A. Generally, you will go through periods of hunger but they will pass, especially if you engage in distracting activities (such as a walk around the neighborhood or chatting with a friend). You really should drink only fresh juice, water, herbal tea, and vegetable broth, but if you are desperate, you can drink some homemade nut milk or vegetables pureed into soup (no dairy added) before continuing on the juice feast as directed. Veering off the cleanse will decrease the cleansing effects, so please do it only if you're absolutely desperate.

Tip: Spiced juice often will quell hunger. I like to add cayenne, ginger, or even jalapeño to my juices. Feel free to experiment.

Q. What if I need to stop the juice feast?

A. If you really need to throw in the towel and break the juice feast, then go for foods that are easy to digest such as light soup, organic rice, or fresh fruit. This is extremely important because you will shock your digestive system if you try to eat anything heavy, and you could end up with stomach pains, cramps, a headache, and major discomfort. How do I know? Because I have done it, and my clients have done it. It's not something you want to experience. I promise.

Even if you stop the juice feast, don't stop the cleanse! Jump right into the next portion of the cleanse, the kidney cleanse food plan. You can still reap benefits.

Q. Why don't the juices contain more fruit?

A. Fruit juice contains sugar and can cause blood sugar imbalances in the body. This can make juice feasting much more difficult and may needlessly stress the body. Furthermore, some people may be dealing with pathogens (viruses, bacteria, fungi such as candida) or parasites that feed on the sugars in the fruit, so it is best to stick with sweet vegetables and low-sugar fruits to sweeten the juice (see shopping list on page 213 for good fruit options).

Q. Can I chew gum during the juice feast?

A. No. Chewing gum activates the digestive enzymes in the body, which interferes with the cleansing process. Furthermore, chewing gum can make you hungry, which is not what you want when you are not eating food.

Q. Can I drink soda, carbonated water, kombucha, or other drinks while juice feasting?

A. Sorry to say, the answer is no. You want to eliminate any distraction from the cleansing process, and carbonation, caffeine, and sugar inhibit this process.

Q. If I do not have a juicer, can I use a blender during the juice feast?

A. Yes, you can use a blender, but purchase cheesecloth or a nut milk bag and strain the pulp. This way you can still take advantage of the juice without the pulp, which contains fiber. Fiber engages the digestive system and slows down the transfer of nutrients, making it less beneficial for our purposes during the juice feast.

If you find that you cannot get enough juice using your type of blender, you can do the cleanse with blended vegetables. While this is not ideal, it will still help you reach your goals.

Q. Why do my smoothies taste grainy?

A. Unfortunately, this is a drawback of many blenders. Without a high-speed motor or the correct blade design, a blender is unable to perfectly blend many ingredients including nuts, vegetables, and fruits. While the graininess isn't harmful and doesn't decrease the nutrient value, it can be less palatable. I love my Vitamix because whatever I blend comes out as smooth as yogurt, and to me that is worth the investment every time.

Q. Can I do just the diet and the cleansing tea without the juice feast?

A. Absolutely. The 3-day juice feast has been designed to jump-start the detoxification process and to stimulate the release of toxins, as well as promote the beneficial physiological changes in the body. However, you can still get great results with just the food plan and tea.

Q. If I know I am not allergic to wheat, soy, and dairy, do I still have to eliminate them during the cleanse?

A. Yes. While you may not be allergic to them, they still can lead to toxic accumulation in the body. The purpose of this cleanse is to reduce the overall toxic load of the body, which includes the elimination of new toxin intake.

It is very important to keep the diet as clean as possible so that the kidneys can focus on clearing waste.

Q. Since the diet eliminates animal products, how am I going to get enough protein?

A. Protein comes from many foods, not just animal products. Plant-based foods are rich in protein, so it's easy to get the recommended requirements. To calculate your daily protein needs in grams, multiple your weight in kilograms by 0.9. (Your weight in pounds divided by 2.2 equals your weight in kilograms.) You will be getting protein from nuts, seeds, beans, grains, and greens. I also recommend that you add a vegan protein powder to your morning smoothie. The best choices are sprouted brown rice, hemp, pea, and chia. See my brand recommendations on page 210.

Q. I have high blood pressure. Should I be consuming sea salt?

A. That depends on how much sea salt you are consuming and what your blood pressure levels are. In general, eliminating sodium of any kind is recommended. However, if you consume very small amounts of sea salt and work with your doctor to monitor your blood pressure, you may be able to include salt in your diet. Sea salt may be able to help normalize blood pressure by balancing minerals, but I have seen this only clinically, not in studies. Therefore, err on the side of caution, start with minimal amounts, and work your way up while under the guidance of your doctor.

Q. Why is potato juice incorporated in the cleanse?

A. Potato juice naturally contains potassium citrate, which countless studies have shown counteracts kidney stone formation. Citrate binds to calcium in the urine, preventing the calcium from binding to oxalate or phosphate. This prevents the accumulation of "gravel," the material that develops into kidney stones. In addition, potassium citrate helps promote an alkaline urine, which also prevents the development of certain kidney stones, such as those composed of uric acid. Potassium citrate is a standard recommendation for kidney stone prevention in both Western and Eastern medical practices.

Q. What type of potato is best for juicing?

A. I suggest using only organic russet potatoes. Make sure that they are not green or sprouting, and feel firm. It is necessary to scrub the potatoes thoroughly, peel them and take out any green sprouts before juicing.

Q. I am doing the 3-day juice feast at a juice store. What juice do I use?
A. Ideally you should bring the recipes from the book and see if the juice store will make them for you. If they are unable, find the juices that most closely match those from the recipes. You can also bring the kidney food guide and make your juices based on that.

Q. I don't have kidney stones. Will this cleanse still be effective for me?
A. Absolutely. The kidneys can accumulate gravel, which may develop into stones. Clearing this material is vital in preventing stones. Gravel isn't something that you feel, but if you have a diet history that includes red meat, soda, caffeine, or vitamin C (ascorbic acid) supplements and you are chronically dehydrated, then there is a good chance you have gravel. This cleanse is focused on prevention, including preventing gravel from turning into stones.

Q. I have a history of kidney stones. Is it really necessary to cleanse my kidneys if the stones have passed?
A. Yes, yes, and yes. If you have had kidney stones in the past, then the chance of recurrence is as high as 75%. A history of stones increases your risk of kidney disease, something that should not be taken lightly. The cleanse is essential to prevention. It is very important that you modify the food plan based on the type of kidney stones you have passed. See the section on kidney stones on page 34.

Q. I have a history of calcium oxalate kidney stones. Why shouldn't I reduce my intake of calcium?
A. The theory that a high consumption of calcium foods leads to the development of calcium kidney stones is now widely recognized as incorrect. Therefore, your consumption of these foods is not restricted.

Q. I have heard that greens have high levels of oxalates? Don't they lead to kidney stones?
A. Yes, greens do contain oxalates, but unless you have a history of calcium oxalate kidney stones, you do not have to worry about it. Research indicates that a large proportion of oxalates accumulated in the body don't come from food (the oxalates in food are not highly absorbable), but rather from internal sources. Also, the degree to which your body absorbs oxalates varies and depends on factors such as gut bacteria colonies, bowel inflammation, and general health. If you do not have a clinical condition in which abnormal

levels of oxalates accumulate, I would not be concerned. But, of course, you can always follow this maxim: everything in moderation.

Q. I feel amazing! How often can I do the cleanse?
A. Great news! You can stay on the kidney cleanse food plan indefinitely because it supplies all the nutrients you need — plus it benefits the whole body and not just the kidneys. As for the juice feast, some people find it beneficial to do it for a day every month, the only caution being that it can result in too much weight loss. But for a general cleansing schedule specific to your needs, see the chapter "After the Cleanse" on page 109.

Q. I feel great, so is there any reason to do another kidney cleanse in the future?
A. I recommend that you continue cleansing your detoxification organs because you are constantly exposed to more toxins than your body can handle. If you follow the health guidelines in this book, do not have any kidney symptoms, and are not in the high-risk group for kidney disease, then performing a kidney cleanse once every few years will suffice. But for every risk factor you have, you will have to re-evaluate the frequency of your cleanse. See the chapter "After the Cleanse" for details.

Q. I did not feel any different on the cleanse and I am still dealing with kidney issues. What should I do?
A. This cleanse is not meant to treat any disease but rather was designed to support the body's natural ability to heal itself, so you may need to continue on the cleanse for longer than the allocated month. A month is merely a general recommendation. Since everyone has different levels of kidney function and toxicity, some people may need to follow the cleanse longer. In addition, if you have not been using the recommended supplements and herbs, I urge you to start now. Sometimes it takes more therapeutic measures, such as the targeted nutrition from these supplements and herbs, to see results.

Another possibility is that there is something else causing kidney stress that you have yet to identify or was not targeted during the cleanse. One situation that I have seen clinically is the role of scars and traumas — such as tailbone injuries, whiplash, episiotomies, C-sections, and other injuries to the back, pelvis, and head — sedating the energy pathways, or meridians, to an organ or gland system. As a result, toxins can more easily accumulate, disconnecting the normal energy flow throughout the body. The only permanent way to resolve the issue is by reopening these meridians through treatment of the scar or trauma. In my clinical practice, the only treatment that has been successful in these cases is the topical use of therapeutic mud, pelotherapy. You can learn more about "mud packing" and find a licensed practitioner by contacting Quantum Nutrition Labs (see page 212).

Q. I suspect that I have heavy metal toxicity. What should I do?
A. Consult a trained practitioner or doctor who can guide you through a heavy metal detoxification program. The kidneys are especially sensitive to heavy metals and can easily be damaged by them, so practicing safe cleansing is very important. Unfortunately, a misguided heavy metal cleanse can harm the body. And please do not use an over-the-counter heavy metal cleansing program — it too can cause harm.

It is also important to eliminate the source of your heavy metal exposure. For example, if you have mercury amalgams (dental fillings), I suggest visiting a biologic dentist who has been trained in safely replacing these fillings.

SPECIFIC NUTRIENT ELIMINATION GUIDE

As you have learned, the kidneys regulate important minerals, such as phosphorus, potassium, and sodium, in the body. When the kidneys begin to fail, they are unable to keep these minerals in balance, making it important for you to control your consumption of foods containing them. If you are dealing with a kidney condition that requires you to eliminate a certain nutrient, you can still follow the kidney cleanse food plan, but you will have to eliminate any foods detrimental to your condition.

PHOSPHORUS AND CHRONIC KIDNEY DISEASE

A person with kidney impairment progressively loses the ability to excrete phosphorus. The body cannot get rid of excess phosphorus and it cannot take in enough calcium to balance the phosphorus. To try and correct this imbalance, the body will "steal" calcium from the bones, weakening them. Thus, cutting back on foods high in phosphorus is highly recommended.

In general, protein-rich foods like meats, milk, eggs, and grains are naturally high in phosphorus and represent the main sources of dietary phosphorus. However, there are now hidden ways in which phosphates are being added to the food supply, which makes it even more important to pay attention to the foods you are consuming.

WHERE ARE PHOSPHATES HIDING?

If eliminating or reducing the foods that contain phosphorus wasn't a hard enough task, now phosphates are hiding in foods that naturally do not contain it. They are being added to a large and increasing number of processed foods, including meats, cheeses, salad dressings, beverages, and bakery products in the form of additives, which are not included in the nutrition facts on the label. Studies have shown that processed meat and poultry products may contain additives that increase phosphorus and potassium content by twofold or threefold, making it even more vital to eliminate these foods.

Calcium-fortified foods are another hidden source of phosphorus because the source of calcium used in these foods is actually calcium phosphate. Foods that typically do not contain calcium, such as orange juice, breads, and breakfast cereals, are now being fortified, making them a new hidden source of phosphorus.

ARE ALL PHOSPHORUS-CONTAINING FOODS ABSORBED EQUALLY?

Reducing your phosphorus intake is not as simple as eliminating foods that contain phosphorus, because the body does not absorb phosphorus from foods equally. For example, phosphorus in additives, preservatives, and sodas are extremely well absorbed by the body (about 90%), whereas phosphorus in plant protein has a lower absorption rate (about 40 to 50%). The phosphorus found in animal protein is more readily absorbed than that in plant protein, making the reduction of animal protein necessary to reduce overall phosphorus intake. The higher the rate of phosphorus absorption a food has, the more important it is to reduce that food.

IS IT POSSIBLE TO FOLLOW THE KIDNEY CLEANSE FOOD PLAN WHILE LOWERING PHOSPHORUS LEVELS?

The great thing about the food plan is that it already eliminates the majority of foods that will raise your phosphorus level. Still, it is important to be aware of the foods allowed on the cleanse that may be high in phosphorus. For those dealing with chronic kidney disease or dialysis, the reduction of these foods may be a permanent change necessary in managing your condition.

HIGH-PHOSPHORUS FOODS

- Beans and lentils
- Beer
- Chocolate
- Cola drinks
- Dairy
- Meat
- Nuts
- Peanut butter
- Poultry
- Processed meats

Avoid foods that contain the following preservatives:

- Dicalcium phosphate
- Hexametaphosphate
- Monocalcium phosphate
- Phosphoric acid
- Polyphosphate
- Pyrophosphate
- Sodium phosphate

Note: While on the kidney cleanse, you can still eat some foods that contain phosphorus, but in moderation. The following are recommended portions.

- Beans and lentils: ½ cup, cooked
- Nuts: ¼ cup

SODIUM

Sodium is one of the most well-known causes of kidney stress, especially in people dealing with high blood pressure or kidney disease. Sodium can cause blood pressure to increase and fluid to build up to unsafe levels when the kidneys aren't functioning properly. Therefore, it is important to avoid foods with more than 100 grams of sodium per serving. Limiting highly processed, canned, smoked, and cured foods is vital since these foods tend to be among the highest in sodium.

During the kidney cleanse, table salt and processed foods rich in sodium are out, but you will be using unheated sea salt. Although sea salt is extremely important for kidney health, it may not be advisable for you if you are dealing with a kidney disorder. Talk to your doctor, who may advise that you refrain from using any salt, even sea salt.

HIGH-SODIUM FOODS

- Canned foods (beans, vegetables)
- Canned or dried soup
- Frozen meals
- Processed cheese
- Salt: table salt, sea salt, seasoned salt
- Salted snack foods
- Soy sauce, miso

POTASSIUM

Now this one really breaks my heart. Some of the healthiest foods for the body contain potassium, but when the kidneys have reached a certain level of dysfunction, potassium restriction becomes necessary.

HIGH-POTASSIUM FOODS

- Apricots
- Artichokes
- Avocados
- Bananas
- Beets
- Brussels sprouts
- Cantaloupe, honeydew melon
- Grapefruit, grapefruit juice
- Greens: collard greens, dandelion greens, mustard greens, chard
- Kiwifruit
- Nectarines
- Oranges, orange juice
- Pears
- Plantains
- Potatoes, sweet potatoes
- Prune juice
- Pumpkin
- Spinach
- Tomato juice, vegetable juice
- Tomatoes
- Winter squash

OXALATES

Oxalates are naturally occurring organic acids. They are created by our own metabolic processes, but also can be absorbed from certain foods. For the majority of us, the consumption of oxalates, especially in moderation, causes no problem. However, if you have a history of calcium oxalate kidney stones, then reducing your intake is advisable. The general recommendation is to limit your intake to 40 to 50 mg each day. This will help reduce the risk of calcium oxalate buildup and potentially the formation of new kidney stones.

VERY HIGH–OXALATE FOODS
(AVOID COMPLETELY: OVER 50 MG/SERVING)

- Almonds
- Beets
- Buckwheat flour
- Miso
- Rhubarb
- Sesame seeds
- Spinach
- Swiss chard
- Tahini

HIGH-OXALATE FOODS
(EAT SPARINGLY: 10–50 MG/SERVING)

- Barley
- Beans: chili, black, great northern, navy, white
- Black pepper
- Black tea
- Breakfast cereals (bran, cream of wheat, granola, grits, raisin bran, shredded wheat)
- Cashews
- Chocolate, cocoa
- Collard greens
- Figs
- Hazelnuts (filberts)
- Kiwifruit
- Lime and lemon peel
- Mustard greens
- Oatmeal
- Okra
- Parsley
- Peanuts, peanut butter
- Pecans
- Peppers (green and chile)
- Potatoes (baked, fried, boiled)
- Rice flour
- Soy (all forms)
- Sweet potatoes
- Wheat flour, wheat germ
- Cornmeal
- Tomatoes, canned or paste

HIGH-METHIONINE FOODS

- Brazil nuts
- Dairy
- Eggs
- Fish (including shellfish)
- Meats (all), including beef, lamb, bison, pork, elk
- Parmesan cheese
- Poultry

- Sesame seeds
- Soy (all forms)
- Sunflower seeds

HIGH-CYSTEINE FOODS

- Broccoli
- Brussels sprouts
- Dairy
- Egg yolks
- Garlic
- Onions
- Oats
- Poultry
- Red bell peppers
- Wheat germ

HIGH-PURINE FOODS

- Anchovies
- Beer (from yeast)
- Game meats
- Herring
- Mackerel
- Organ meats
- Sardines
- Scallops
- Sweetbreads

MODERATE-PURINE FOODS

- Asparagus
- Beef
- Cauliflower
- Fish and seafood (besides those listed in "High-Purine Foods")
- Legumes
- Oatmeal
- Pork
- Poultry
- Mushrooms
- Wheat bran and germ

KITCHEN CABINET CLEANUP

One of the keys to success on the kidney cleanse is making sure that your home is set up to be your biggest supporter, not your taunting opponent. The foods in your kitchen should be kidney cleanse–approved, so even at your weakest moment there will be nothing for you to cheat with. I have put together a list of pantry items so you can restock your cabinets for success. Making sure you don't have items containing nasty fillers and additives could be a full-time job—so sticking to this list is the easiest route!

Cleanse your kitchen, just as you will your kidneys, by removing foods containing these toxic ingredients. Check labels carefully.

- High-fructose corn syrup
- Partially hydrogenated oils
- Polyunsaturated oils (trans fatty acids)
- Shortening and canola oil
- Monosodium glutamate (MSG)
- Natural flavors or spices (MSG)
- Sodium or potassium benzoate
- Nitrates
- Food colors and dyes
- Polysorbate 60
- Modified corn starch
- Sodium aluminum sulfate

KITCHEN CABINET ESSENTIALS

(Organic, GMO-free)

Condiments

- Balsamic vinegar
- Brown rice vinegar
- Coconut oil, unrefined
- Minced ginger
- Miso
- Nama shoyu (unpasteurized soy sauce)
- Nutritional yeast
- Olive oil, extra-virgin (in a dark bottle)
- Sea salt, unrefined

Canned and jarred goods

- Canned tomatoes (no high-fructose corn syrup)
- Kalamata olives
- Ketchup (no high-fructose corn syrup)
- Pasta sauce
- Roasted peppers
- Sun-dried tomatoes
- Vegetable broth (free of canola oil)

Healthy grains

- Breakfast grains (quinoa, buckwheat, gluten-free oatmeal, whole oat groats)
- Exotic rice (forbidden black or basmati)
- Germinated brown rice
- Quinoa pasta
- Sprouted corn tortillas (GMO-free)
- Sprouted quinoa

Beans and legumes

- Black beans
- Bulk bin lima beans
- Canned beans and lentils (BPA-free cans)
- Cannellini beans
- Sprouted green lentils

Nuts and seeds

- Sprouted nuts and seeds
- Unheated, unroasted, and unsalted raw nut butter (no peanut butter)

Sweet stuff

- Coconut flakes, organic
- Coconut sugar
- Dried fruits (sulfur-free, no added sugar and oil)
- Goji berries
- Grade B or #2 maple syrup
- Honey, raw
- Molasses

Snack stuff

- Kale chips
- Raw flax and vegetable crackers
- Raw food bars
- Seed crackers, gluten-free

Baking items

- Flour and wheat alternatives (coconut, almonds, brown rice)
- Gluten-free baking mixes
- Baking soda (aluminum-free)
- Coconut butter
- Vanilla extract

RESOURCES

Before you start the cleanse, I encourage you to check out these highly recommended websites and books. Many of the resources I've listed feature delicious recipes. While this book has wonderful recipes, you may want to look to these other books and websites for variety.

Note: Not all the recipes on the websites use kidney cleanse–approved foods, but you can modify them by substituting the approved foods from this book.

HEALTH BOOKS

Animal, Vegetable, Miracle by Barbara Kingsolver
Cooked by Michael Pollan
Diet for a Hot Planet: The Climate Crisis by Anna Lappé
Eating for Beauty by David Wolfe
Eating Well for Optimum Health by Dr. Andrew Weil, M.D.
8 Weeks to Optimum Health by Dr. Andrew Weil, M.D.
Fast Food Nation by Eric Schlosser
Food, Inc. edited by Karl Weber
Food Rules: An Eater's Manual by Michael Pollan
Healthy Aging by Dr. Andrew Weil, M.D.
In Defense of Food by Michael Pollan
The Omnivore's Dilemma by Michael Pollan
Superfoods: The Food and Medicine of the Future by David Wolfe

COOKBOOKS

The Adaptable Feast by Ivy Manning
Ani's Raw Food Essentials by Ani Phyo
Candle 79 by Joy Pierson, Angel Ramos, and Jorge Pineda
Chloe's Kitchen by Chloe Coscarelli
Clean Food by Terry Walters
The Conscious Cook by Tal Ronnen
Earth to Table by Jeff Crump and Bettina Schormann
Everyday Raw by Matthew Kenney
The Green Kitchen by David Frenkiel and Luise Vindahl
Herbivoracious by Michael Natkin
The Kind Diet by Alicia Silverstone
La Tartine Gourmande by Beatrice Peltre
Love Soup by Anna Thomas
The Modern Vegetarian by Maria Elia
Plenty by Yotam Ottolenghi
Practically Raw by Amber Shea Crawley
Pure Vegan by Joseph Shuldiner
Quinoa 365 by Patricia Green and Carolyn Hemming
Raw: The UNcook book by Juliano
RAWvolution by Matt Amsden
The Real Food Daily Cookbook by Ann Gentry
Small Plates and Sweet Treats by Aran Goyoaga
The Sprouted Kitchen by Sara Forte and High Forte
Super Natural Every Day by Heidi Swanson
Superfood Kitchen by Julie Morris
Superfood Smoothies by Julie Morris
Vegetarian Everyday by David Frenkiel and Luise Vindahl

HEALTH MOVIES

Crazy Sexy Cancer
Fast Food Nation
Fat, Sick & Nearly Dead
Food Matters
Forks Over Knives
Fresh

The Gerson Miracle
Hungry for Change
Ingredients
May I Be Frank
Osmosis Jones (great for children)
Simply Raw
Tapped

RECIPE WEBSITES

www.101cookbooks.com
www.greenkitchenstories.com
www.sproutedkitchen.com
www.thefirstmess.com
www.mynewroots.org
www.umamigirl.com
www.roostblog.com
www.purevege.com
www.loveandlemons.com

OTHER WEBSITES

www.ted.com (TED Talks)
www.thechalkboardmag.com
www.mercola.com
www.drweil.com
www.care2.com
www.mindbodygreen.com
www.onegreenplanet.org
www.extremehealthradio.com
www.oneradionetwork.com
www.qnlabs.com (Healthline radio)

JUICE BARS

If you are unable to make your own juice at home for the 3-day juice feast and want to go to a local juice bar instead, please choose a place that makes juice fresh daily or uses a hydraulic press juicer. Juice made with a hydraulic press is often referred to as "pressed juice." The following are among the acceptable juice bars.

Earthbar

Juice Crafters

Franklin Juice Company

JuiceLand

Kreation Organic Juicery

Moon Juice

Nekter Juice Bar

Pressed Juicery

Whole Foods Market (locations with juice bars)

PRODUCT RECOMMENDATIONS

The following are my favorite products and suppliers. Use them during the cleanse and afterward to keep your kidneys happy, healthy, and toxin-free.

KIDNEY TEA

Dandelion Leaf Tea and Corn Silk Loose Herbs or Extract

Mountain Rose Herbs

P.O. Box 50220, Eugene, OR 97405

(800) 879-3337

International: (541) 741-7307

www.mountainroseherbs.com

Celebration Herbals

33230 Pettit Rd Wainfleet, ON, Canada

celebrationherbals.com

PROTEIN POWDER

Epic Protein

Sprout Living

(888) 633-5984

www.sproutliving.com

Hemp Protein

Manitoba Harvest

(800) 665-4367

www.manitobaharvest.com

Nutiva Hemp Protein
(800) 993-4367
www.nutiva.com

Perfect Fit Protein
Tone It Up
my.toneitup.com

Raw Protein
Garden of Life
866-465-0051
www.gardenoflife.com

Vega One Performance Protein
Vega
(866) 839-8863
www.myvega.com

Warrior Blend (pea, cranberry, hemp)
Classic Protein (sprouted brown rice)
Sunwarrior
(888) 540-3667
www.sunwarrior.com

JUICERS
Centrifugal: Breville, Cuisinart, Omega
Masticating: Omega, Breville, Hurom, Champion
Hydraulic press: Norwalk

HIGH-SPEED BLENDERS
VitaMix
BlendTec

SUPPLEMENTS

Antioxidants
Green Tea PG–Quantum Nutrition Labs
Resveratrol–Quantum Nutrition Labs
Alpha Lipoic Acid–Pure Encapsulations
CoQ10–Pure Encapsulations

Rooibos Powdered Extract–Immunologic

Digestive Agents

HCl–Quantum Nutrition Labs
Digest–Quantum Nutrition Labs
Aloe Ferox–Immunologic

Greens Powders

Greens Mix–Quantum Nutrition Labs
Ormus Supergreens–Sunwarrior
Sweet Wheat–Immunologic

Minerals

Liquid Light–Sunwarrior
Ionic Mineral Drops–Immunologic
pH Salts–Immunologic
Pink Salt–Quantum Nutrition Labs

SUPPLEMENT COMPANIES

Immunologic
(512) 541-4338
www.immunologic.com

Pure Encapsulations
(800) 753-2277
www.pureencapsulations.com

Quantum Nutrition Labs
(800) 370-3447
www.qnlabs.com

Sunwarrior
(888) 540-3667
www.sunwarrior.com

DETOXIFICATION PRODUCTS

CASTOR OIL: Quantum Nutrition Labs, Heritage Products, Home Health

ENEMA BUCKET: Quantum Nutrition Labs

FOOT SOAKS AND EXTERNAL MUD: Medi-Bath, Medi-Soak, Medi-Magma
by Quantum Nutrition Labs

NETI POT: Himalayan Institute, Ancient Secrets, Surthrival (Daniel Vitalis)

KIDNEY CLEANSE SHOPPING LIST

KIDNEY-FRIENDLY FOODS AND SUPERFOODS

- ☐ Apple cider vinegar
- ☐ Asparagus
- ☐ Beets
- ☐ Black cherries
- ☐ Black maca
- ☐ Black sesame seeds
- ☐ Black walnuts
- ☐ Cayenne
- ☐ Celery
- ☐ Cranberry
- ☐ Cucumber
- ☐ Dandelion
- ☐ Flaxseeds
- ☐ Green tea
- ☐ Lemon
- ☐ Lime
- ☐ Parsley
- ☐ Peppermint
- ☐ Potato juice
- ☐ Turmeric
- ☐ Watermelon

SUPERFOOD SUPPLEMENTS

- ☐ Acai
- ☐ Bee pollen
- ☐ Camu camu
- ☐ Chlorella
- ☐ Goji berries
- ☐ Lucuma powder
- ☐ Spirulina

FRUITS

- ☐ Apple
- ☐ Apricot
- ☐ Blackberry
- ☐ Blueberry
- ☐ Boysenberry
- ☐ Cherry
- ☐ Coconut
- ☐ Cranberry
- ☐ Elderberry
- ☐ Gooseberry
- ☐ Grapefruit
- ☐ Kiwi
- ☐ Lemon
- ☐ Lime
- ☐ Loganberry
- ☐ Nectarine
- ☐ Peach
- ☐ Pear
- ☐ Plum
- ☐ Raspberry
- ☐ Rhubarb
- ☐ Strawberry

HIGH SUGAR

- ☐ Banana
- ☐ Cantaloupe
- ☐ Date
- ☐ Dried currant
- ☐ Dried fig
- ☐ Fig
- ☐ Grape
- ☐ Guava
- ☐ Honeydew melon
- ☐ Lychee
- ☐ Mango
- ☐ Papaya
- ☐ Persimmon
- ☐ Pineapple
- ☐ Pomegranate
- ☐ Prune
- ☐ Raisin
- ☐ Watermelon

SEA VEGETABLES

- ☐ Agar
- ☐ Arame
- ☐ Dulse
- ☐ Hijiki
- ☐ Irish moss

- ☐ Kelp
- ☐ Kombu
- ☐ Laver
- ☐ Nori
- ☐ Wakame

VEGETABLES

- ☐ Arugula
- ☐ Beet greens
- ☐ Cilantro
- ☐ Collard greens
- ☐ Dandelion greens
- ☐ Endive
- ☐ Kale
- ☐ Lettuce
- ☐ Mustard greens
- ☐ Parsley
- ☐ Radicchio
- ☐ Spinach
- ☐ Sprouts
- ☐ Swiss chard
- ☐ Turnip greens
- ☐ Watercress

MEDIUM STARCH

- ☐ Avocado
- ☐ Bamboo shoots
- ☐ Bok choy
- ☐ Daikon
- ☐ Eggplant
- ☐ Fennel
- ☐ Green beans
- ☐ Jicama
- ☐ Leeks
- ☐ Okra
- ☐ Olives
- ☐ Peppers (bell)
- ☐ Radishes
- ☐ Turnips
- ☐ Water chestnuts
- ☐ Zucchini

LOW STARCH

- ☐ Asparagus
- ☐ Broccoli
- ☐ Brussels sprouts
- ☐ Cabbage
- ☐ Cauliflower
- ☐ Celery
- ☐ Cucumber
- ☐ Garlic
- ☐ Gingerroot
- ☐ Mushrooms
- ☐ Onions
- ☐ Peppers (hot)
- ☐ Scallions
- ☐ Shallots

HIGH STARCH

- ☐ Artichokes
- ☐ Beets
- ☐ Carrots
- ☐ Celery root
- ☐ Corn
- ☐ Green peas
- ☐ Parsnip
- ☐ Potato
- ☐ Pumpkin
- ☐ Rutabaga
- ☐ Squash (summer)
- ☐ Squash (winter)
- ☐ Sweet Potato
- ☐ Yam

MUSHROOMS

- ☐ Button
- ☐ Chanterelle
- ☐ Cremini

- ☐ Shiitake
- ☐ Truffle
- ☐ Trumpet

NUTS AND SEEDS (RAW AND SPROUTED)

- ☐ Almonds
- ☐ Brazil nuts
- ☐ Cashews
- ☐ Chestnuts
- ☐ Chia seeds
- ☐ Flaxseeds
- ☐ Hazelnuts
- ☐ Hemp seeds
- ☐ Macadamia nuts
- ☐ Pecans
- ☐ Pine nuts
- ☐ Pistachios
- ☐ Poppy seeds
- ☐ Pumpkin seeds
- ☐ Salba seeds
- ☐ Sesame seeds
- ☐ Sunflower seeds
- ☐ Walnuts

GRAINS (GLUTEN-FREE)

- ☐ Amaranth
- ☐ Basmati rice
- ☐ Black rice
- ☐ Brown rice
- ☐ Buckwheat
- ☐ Corn (non GMO, organic)
- ☐ Millet
- ☐ Quinoa
- ☐ Oats (gluten-free)
- ☐ Teff

PROTEIN

- ☐ Blue green algae powder
- ☐ Legumes (beans; see also Legumes)
- ☐ Mushrooms
- ☐ Nutritional yeast
- ☐ Nuts (raw)
- ☐ Protein powder (vegan)
- ☐ Seeds, raw
- ☐ Tempeh (organic)

LEGUMES

- ☐ Aduki beans
- ☐ Black beans
- ☐ Black-eyed peas
- ☐ Fava beans
- ☐ Garbanzo beans
- ☐ Kidney beans
- ☐ Lentils
- ☐ Lima beans
- ☐ Mung beans
- ☐ Navy beans
- ☐ Pinto beans
- ☐ White beans

FATS AND OILS

- ☐ Almond oil
- ☐ Avocado oil
- ☐ Black currant oil
- ☐ Black truffle oil
- ☐ Borage oil
- ☐ Cacao butter
- ☐ Coconut butter
- ☐ Coconut oil
- ☐ Flaxseed oil
- ☐ Grapeseed oil
- ☐ Hazelnut oil
- ☐ Hemp oil
- ☐ Nut butter (raw)
- ☐ Olive oil (extra virgin)
- ☐ Pumpkin seed oil
- ☐ Sesame oil
- ☐ Walnut oil
- ☐ Wheat germ oil

HERBS AND SPICES

- ☐ Anise
- ☐ Basil
- ☐ Bay leaf
- ☐ Caraway
- ☐ Cayenne
- ☐ Chili powder
- ☐ Chive
- ☐ Cilantro
- ☐ Cinnamon
- ☐ Clove
- ☐ Coriander
- ☐ Cumin
- ☐ Curry powder
- ☐ Dill weed
- ☐ Fennel
- ☐ Fenugreek
- ☐ Ginger
- ☐ Mace
- ☐ Marjoram
- ☐ Mint
- ☐ Mustard seed
- ☐ Nutmeg
- ☐ Oregano
- ☐ Paprika
- ☐ Parsley
- ☐ Pepper
- ☐ Peppermint
- ☐ Rosemary
- ☐ Saffron
- ☐ Sage
- ☐ Savory
- ☐ Spearmint
- ☐ Tarragon
- ☐ Thyme
- ☐ Turmeric

SWEETENERS

- ☐ Coconut nectar
- ☐ Coconut sugar
- ☐ Date syrup
- ☐ Dates
- ☐ Figs
- ☐ Honey (raw)
- ☐ Maples syrup (grade B)
- ☐ Molasses
- ☐ Stevia
- ☐ Yacon syrup

CONDIMENTS

- Apple cider vinegar
- Balsamic vinegar
- Brown rice vinegar
- Coconut vinegar
- Garlic powder
- Horse radish
- Hot sauce
- Lemon juice
- Miso (organic)
- Mustard
- Nutritional yeast
- Olive oil (extra virgin)
- Red wine vinegar
- Sea salt (unrefined)
- Soy sauce substitute
- Vanilla beans/extract
- Wasabi

BEVERAGES

- Almond milk
- Coconut milk/kefir
- Coconut water
- Filtered water (reverse-osmosis)
- Fruit juice (fresh-pressed)
- Hemp milk
- Herbal tea (loose-leaf is best)
- Oat milk
- Rice milk
- Vegetable juice (fresh)

DRIED GOODS

- Almond flour
- Buckwheat flour
- Buckwheat noodles
- Canned beans (organic)
- Canned rice (organic)
- Canned tomato sauce (organic)
- Canned tomatoes (organic)
- Coconut flakes
- Coconut flour
- Crackers (gluten-free)
- Crackers (raw)
- Granola (raw)
- Hemp flour
- Kale chips (raw)
- Oat flour
- Pasta, brown rice
- Pasta, quinoa
- Quinoa flour
- Raw food nutrition bars
- Sprouted grains/beans/lentils
- Trail mix (raw)
- Vegetable stock

OTHER (JARRED ITEMS)

- Artichoke hearts
- Capers
- Coconut yogurt
- Kimchi
- Nut butter (raw)
- Olives
- Pickles
- Roasted peppers
- Salsa
- Sauerkraut
- Sun-dried tomatoes

FROZEN GOODS

- ❏ Frozen fruit (for smoothies)
- ❏ Frozen vegetables
- ❏ Gluten-free bread
- ❏ Gluten-free tortillas

DESSERTS (CHOCOLATE/CACAO FREE)

- ❏ Blended fruit "ice cream"
- ❏ Dried fruit (dates, figs)
- ❏ Fresh fruit Popsicles
- ❏ Ice cream (coconut, cashew, or hemp milk)
- ❏ Raw desserts

ORGANIC/CONVENTIONAL SHOPPING LIST

MUST BE PURCHASED ORGANIC

- ❏ Apples
- ❏ Celery
- ❏ Cherry tomatoes
- ❏ Cucumbers
- ❏ Grapes
- ❏ Hot peppers
- ❏ Kale/collard greens
- ❏ Nectarines
- ❏ Peaches
- ❏ Potatoes
- ❏ Spinach
- ❏ Strawberries
- ❏ Summer squash
- ❏ Sweet bell peppers

CAN BE PURCHASED CONVENTIONAL

- ❏ Asparagus
- ❏ Avocado
- ❏ Cabbage
- ❏ Cantaloupe (domestic)
- ❏ Eggplant
- ❏ Grapefruit
- ❏ Kiwi
- ❏ Mangoes
- ❏ Mushrooms
- ❏ Onions
- ❏ Papayas
- ❏ Pineapples
- ❏ Sweet corn
- ❏ Sweet peas
- ❏ Sweet potatoes

KIDNEY-WEAKENING FOODS (ELIMINATED ON THE CLEANSE)

GLUTEN GRAINS

- ☐ Barley
- ☐ Bran
- ☐ Bulgur
- ☐ Couscous
- ☐ Farina
- ☐ Farro
- ☐ Graham
- ☐ Kamut
- ☐ Male
- ☐ Malt
- ☐ Matza
- ☐ Oats
- ☐ Rye
- ☐ Seitan
- ☐ Semolina
- ☐ Spelt
- ☐ Wheat
- ☐ Wheat flour
- ☐ Wheat germ
- ☐ Wheat protein
- ☐ Wheat starch

CARBONATED BEVERAGES

- ☐ Soda/cola
- ☐ Soda water
- ☐ Sparkling water
- ☐ Tonic water

UNFERMENTED SOY

- ☐ Bean curd
- ☐ Edamame
- ☐ Hydrolyzed soy protein
- ☐ Soy butter
- ☐ Soy cheese
- ☐ Soy ice cream
- ☐ Soy nuts
- ☐ Soy protein
- ☐ Soy whipped cream
- ☐ Soy yogurt
- ☐ Soybean oil
- ☐ Soymilk
- ☐ Textured soy flour
- ☐ Textured vegetable protein
- ☐ Tofu

ARTIFICIAL SWEETENERS

- ☐ Acesulfame K
- ☐ Aspartame
- ☐ Equal
- ☐ NutraSweet
- ☐ Saccharin
- ☐ Splenda
- ☐ Sucralose
- ☐ Sweet One
- ☐ Sweet'N Low

SODIUM-RICH FOODS

(check labels for less than 140 mg/serving)

- ☐ Bouillon cubes
- ☐ Boxed foods
- ☐ Boxed rice dinners
- ☐ Canned foods
- ☐ Canned soup
- ☐ Chips
- ☐ Condiments
- ☐ Convenience foods
- ☐ Frozen dinners
- ☐ Garlic salt
- ☐ Popcorn
- ☐ Prepackaged snacks
- ☐ Salad dressing
- ☐ Salted nuts
- ☐ Salted pretzels
- ☐ Table salt

ANIMAL PROTEIN

- ☐ Beef
- ☐ Cured meats
- ☐ Eggs
- ☐ Fish
- ☐ Lamb
- ☐ Pork
- ☐ Poultry
- ☐ Shellfish
- ☐ Veal

DAIRY

- ☐ Butter
- ☐ Buttermilk
- ☐ Casein
- ☐ Cheese
- ☐ Cream
- ☐ Cream cheese
- ☐ Creamer
- ☐ Crème fraîche
- ☐ Half-and-half
- ☐ Ice cream
- ☐ Kefir
- ☐ Lactose
- ☐ Milk
- ☐ Pudding
- ☐ Sour cream
- ☐ Whey
- ☐ Whipped cream
- ☐ Yogurt

CAFFEINE

- ☐ Chocolate
- ☐ Coffee
- ☐ Espresso
- ☐ Energy drinks
- ☐ Non-herbal tea
- ☐ Soda
- ☐ Workout powders

ALCOHOL

- ☐ Beer
- ☐ Hard cider
- ☐ Liqueurs
- ☐ Sake
- ☐ Sparkling wine
- ☐ Spirits
- ☐ Wine

PROTEIN POWDERS

- ☐ Casein
- ☐ Egg white
- ☐ Soy
- ☐ Whey

REFINED SUGAR

- ☐ Barley malt syrup
- ☐ Brown sugar
- ☐ Cane sugar/juice
- ☐ Corn syrup
- ☐ Dextrin
- ☐ Dextrose
- ☐ Fructose
- ☐ Glucose
- ☐ High-fructose corn syrup
- ☐ Honey (not raw)
- ☐ Malt syrup
- ☐ Maltodextrin
- ☐ Maltose
- ☐ Raw sugar
- ☐ Rice syrup
- ☐ Sucrose
- ☐ Turbinado sugar
- ☐ White sugar

OTHER

- ☐ Creatine

WHAT TO WATCH OUT FOR

- ☐ Bagels
- ☐ Breads
- ☐ Breakfast bars
- ☐ Canola oil
- ☐ Cereal
- ☐ Crackers
- ☐ Dough (pizza, pie)
- ☐ Food bars
- ☐ Granola bars
- ☐ Parmesan "cheese"
- ☐ Seitan
- ☐ Soy crisps
- ☐ Soymilk
- ☐ Vegan buttery spread
- ☐ Vegan cheese (Daiya, Dr. Cow, Follow Your Heart)
- ☐ Vegan cream cheese
- ☐ Vegenaise
- ☐ Veggie burgers
- ☐ Veggie deli meat
- ☐ Veggie dogs

NEPHROTOXIC SUBSTANCES

CHEMOTHERAPY AGENTS

- Anti-angiogenesis agents
- Gemcitabine
- Ifosfamide
- Interleukin-2
- Methotrexate
- Mitomycin
- Platins

DIAGNOSTIC AGENTS

- High osmolar
- Iso-osmolar
- Low osmolar

HERBAL REMEDIES

- Aristolochic acid
- Cat's claw
- Chaparral
- Datura sp.
- Ephedra sp.
- Germanium
- Glycyrrhiza sp. (licorice)
- Taxus celebica (Chinese Yew)
- Willow bark
- Wormwood oil
- Yellow oleander

ANALGESICS

- Analgesic combinations
- NSAIDs
- Phenacetin
- Selective COX-2 Inhibitors

HEAVY METALS

- Arsenic
- Bismuth
- Cadmium
- Copper
- Lead
- Mercury
- Uranium

ORGANIC CHEMICALS

- Alachlor
- Dalapon
- Dibromide
- Dichlorobenzene
- Ethylbenzene
- Glyphosate
- Hexachlorobenzene
- Hexachlorocyclopentadiene
- Lindane
- Pentachlorophenol
- Styrene
- Toluene
- Toxaphene
- Trichloroethane

RECREATIONAL DRUGS

☐ Cocaine

IMMUNOSUPPRESSIVES

☐ Calcineurin inhibitors
☐ Sirolimus

ADULTERANTS

☐ Cadmium
☐ Dichromate
☐ Mefenamic acid

☐ Melamine
☐ Phenylbutazone

SOLVENTS

☐ Hydrocarbons

OTHER

☐ ACE inhibitors/ARBs
☐ Antacids
☐ Conjugated estrogens
☐ Cyclosporine
☐ Gadolinium (in high doses)
☐ Getamicin
☐ Hydrazine
☐ Hydroxyethyl starch, mannitol
☐ Indinavir (esp. with TMP-SMX)
☐ Mesalamine
☐ Methoxyflurane

☐ NSAIDs
☐ Oral NaP solution
☐ Orlistat
☐ Pamidronate
☐ Silicon
☐ Statins
☐ Topiramate, zonisamide
☐ Uranium
☐ Yohimbe
☐ Zolendronate

	Meat Products			Dairy Products			
	Day 30	Day 31	Day 32	Day 33	Day 34	Day 35	Day 36
Upon Rising							
Breakfast							
Mid-Morning							
Lunch							
Afternoon							
Dinner							
Before Bedtime							

	Gluten Products		Caffeine			Soy Products	
	Day 37	Day 38	Day 39	Day 40	Day 41	Day 42	Day 43
Upon Rising							
Breakfast							
Mid-Morning							
Lunch							
Afternoon							
Dinner							
Before Bedtime							

CONVERSION CHARTS

VOLUME

U.S.	U.S. EQUIVALENT	METRIC
1 tablespoon / 3 teaspoons	½ fluid ounce	15 ml
¼ cup	2 fluid ounces	60 ml
⅓ cup	3 fluid ounces	90 ml
½ cup	4 fluid ounces	120 ml
⅔ cup	5 fluid ounces	150 ml
¾ cup	6 fluid ounces	180 ml
1 cup	8 fluid ounces	240 ml
2 cups	16 fluid ounces	480 ml

WEIGHT

U.S.	METRIC
½ ounce	15 grams
1 ounce	30 grams
2 ounces	60 grams
¼ pound	115 grams
⅓ pound	150 grams
½ pound	225 grams
¾ pound	350 grams
1 pound	450 grams

INDEX

black foods, 65
black maca, 65
black mushrooms, 65
black sesame cucumber salad, 151
black sesame seeds, 65
black tea, 67
black/tart cherries, 62
black walnuts, 65
blender, 73
blood cleansing, 19–22
blood volume and pressure, 20–21
blueberries, 132
bone loss–pH connection, 55–56
bone marrow, 24–25
bones, 24–25
bowel elimination, basics of, 87–91.
    See also enemas
    constipation, 89
    digestion connection, 89
    magnesium-constipation connec-
        tion, 90–91
BPA-free plastic water, 77
brain, 24–25
brushite, 124–125
Brussels sprouts salad with parsley
    lemon vinaigrette, 157
2-butoxyethanol, 17
butternut squash marinara, 171
Butyl cellosolve, 17
B vitamins, 131

C

cabbage, 65
    and leek soup, 145
cadmium, 15
caffeine, 67
calcium oxalate kidney stones, 195
calcium stones, 124–125
caramelized onion, 187
carbonated beverages, 66
carbon dioxide, 14
cashew blueberry smoothie, 142
cashew parmesan, 173
castor oil, 104–107
    packs, 81, 106–107

catecholamine hormones role,
    101–102
cauliflower cream puree, 184
Cayce, Edgar, 104
cayenne, 63
celery, 63
celery pear juice, 139
centrifugal juicer, 72
ceteareth-20, 12
Chanca Piedra (Phyllanthus niruri),
    127–128
"cheesy" broccoli, 182
"cheesy" collard wraps, 173
"Cheesy Mayo," 186
chemicals, 14–16
    to avoid in household cleaning
        products, 17
    to avoid in personal care
        products, 16
chia seeds, 65
Chinese medicine, 23
Chinese tempeh salad, 158
chlorinated phenols, 17
chlorine, 12
chloroform, 12
chlorophyll, 56
chocolate, 67
chronic kidney disease (CKD), 130,
    133–134, 198–200
cleansing kidneys, 2–3, 36–52, 71–85,
    188–197. See also food plan in
    kidney cleansing; post cleansing
    adjunct therapies, 49, 79, 81–82
    adjusting conditions, 123
    affecting urine pH, 92
    Astragalus (Astragalus
        Membranaceus), 83–84
    basics, 37
    blood sugar and, 191
    breastfeeding and, 188
    concept of, 2
    Cordyceps sinensis, 82–83
    3-day juice feast, 39–42. See also
        juice feasting
    dietary recommendations, 75
    diuretics and, 190

mint mojito protein smoothie, 144
minty green smoothie, 143
morphine (poppy), 43

N

naphthalene, 17
nephrolithiasis, 124–128
    risk factors for, 34–35
nephrons, 18
nephrotoxic substances, 223–226
    adulterants, 224
    analgesics, 223
    chemotherapy agents, 223
    diagnostic agents, 223
    heavy metals, 223
    herbal remedies, 223
    immunosuppressives, 224
    organic chemicals, 223
    recreational drugs, 224
    solvents, 224
nitrobenzene, 17
nonylphenol ethoxylate, 17
nordic harvest salad with lemony
    dressing and superfoods, 161
norepinephrine (noradrenaline), 101
nuts, 65

O

omega-3 fatty acids, 65, 126, 131–132
ongoing cleansing, recommendations
    for, 119–120
    daily practices, 119–120
    weekly practices, 120
orange lassi smoothie, 141
original qi (chi), 23
outdoor air pollution, 12
oxalates, 124–125, 201
    high-oxalate foods, 202
    very high–oxalate foods, 202

P

parabens, 12, 16
para-dichlorobenzene, 17
parasympathetic (kidney-healing)
    state, 95–96
parathyroid connection, 134–136

parathyroid dysfunction, 134–136
parathyroid hormone (PTH), 133
parsley, 63, 65
parsley green smoothie, 145
parsnip sushi rolls, 177
pear juice, 139
peppermint leaves, 63
perchloroethylene, 12, 17
perfluorooctanoic acid, 12
pesto, 175
petrolatum, 16
petroleum distillates/solvents, 17
pH (acid-alkaline) balance, 20
pH Miracle, The, 55
pH of foods and cleansing, 54
    alkalizing foods, 56
    bone loss–pH connection, 55–56
    chronic acidic pH, 56
pH reading, 91–92
    cleansing affecting urine pH, 92
phenol, 16–17
phosphates, 17, 124–125, 199
phosphorus kidney disease, 198–200
phosphorus-containing foods, 199
    high-phosphorus foods, 200
phthalates, 11–12, 16
plant-based diet, 117
plant-based protein, 65
polenta, 175
polycystic kidney disease, 34
polyethoxyethylene mineral oil, 16
polyethylene glycols (PEGs), 12, 16
polyvinyl chloride (PVC), 11
pomegranate eggplant ratatouille, 165
pomegranate Persian kale chips, 179
post cleansing, 109–122. *See also* rein-
    troducing foods
    annual cleanses, 117–120
    diet including animal protein, 118
    healthy eating tenets, 113–115
    high toxic load, 118
    liver/gallbladder and intestinal
        cleansing, 119
    making the right food choices,
        113–115
    plant-based diet, 117

ACKNOWLEDGMENTS

This book was made possible by the influence and love of so many people who have acted as my mentors, angels, and loving supporters. For that I am eternally grateful. With open eyes, ears, mind, and heart, I created this book with the hope that it will contribute a unique perspective on health, one that will provide the guidance so many people need. I was inspired by many brilliant minds and passionate hearts, and I hope that, though this book, I will inspire others to reach happiness and health.

First, I want to thank my family and close friends for supporting my passion and purpose in life, and for instilling in me the hope and unconditional love needed to complete this book. Second, I would like to thank my guardian angels, Elle Nevarde, Joie Felts, Lisa Klinker, and Marjolaine Hebert, for believing in me and providing me with the fearlessness, strength, unwavering faith, and clarity of mind that made my work possible. Third, I want to thank my mentors, Dr. Vincent Medici and Dr. Robert Marshall, for expanding my mind and sharing with me their priceless knowledge and perspectives. Finally, I want to give a special heart-filled thanks to my loving supporters Dr. Austin Chen, Debra Consani, and Hesaam Moallem, who have been my rock and lighthouse during this journey in which the destination and pathways have often remained unknown and unseen.

Thought is the matrix of all creation; thought created everything. If you hold on to that truth with indomitable will, you can materialize any thought.
— Paramahansa Yogananda

Whatever the present moment contains, accept it as if you have chosen it. Always work with it, not against it. Make it your friend and ally, not your enemy. This will miraculously transform your whole life. — Eckhart Tolle

ABOUT THE AUTHOR

LAUREN FELTS is a certified nutritionist who has mastered the art of health through multiple paths of training. After graduating from the University of Southern California, Lauren embarked on a personal journey to improve her own health and broaden her knowledge. She gained expertise in many areas of the wellness field: managing sales and education for a national supplements manufacturer, working with clients in her private practice, contributing editorials to influential publications, and supporting the launch of a raw culinary school and restaurant.